The WORD *of* WISDOM

DISCOVERING THE LDS CODE OF HEALTH

DR. SCOTT A. JOHNSON

CFI

AN IMPRINT OF CEDAR FORT, INC.

SPRINGVILLE, UTAH

ISBN 13: 978-1-4621-1160-2

Published by CFI, an imprint of Cedar Fort, Inc., 2373 W. 700 S., Springville, UT 84663
Distributed by Cedar Fort, Inc., www.cedarfort.com.

LIBRARY OF CONGRESS CATALOGING-IN-PUBLICATION DATA

Johnson, Scott A., 1976- author.
The Word of Wisdom : discovering the LDS code of health / Dr. Scott A. Johnson.
 pages cm
Includes bibliographical references and index.
Summary: Nutritional guidance to help individuals make correct dietary choices.
ISBN 978-1-4621-1160-2 (alk. paper)
1. Word of wisdom. 2. Nutrition--Religious aspects--Church of Jesus Christ of Latter-day Saints.
3. Nutrition--Religious aspects--Mormon Church. 4. Health--Religious aspects--Church of Jesus
Christ of Latter-day Saints. 5. Health--Religious aspects--Mormon Church. 6. Church of Jesus
Christ of Latter-day Saints--Doctrines. 7. Mormon Church--Doctrines. I. Title.

BX8629.W63J64 2013
613.2088'28--dc23

 2012044973

Cover design by Erica Dixon
Cover design © 2013 by Lyle Mortimer
Edited and typeset by Whitney A. Lindsley

Printed in the United States of America

10 9 8 7 6 5 4 3 2 1

Printed on acid-free paper

To my ever-supportive family, especially my wife and children, who made considerable sacrifices for me to write this book. Special thanks to my parents for always championing my books. To my Heavenly Father for providing the inspiration and courage necessary to see this book to its conclusion. And to all those individuals who tirelessly promote healthy nutrition and lifestyle choices—I salute you and wish you abundant health and wellness.

IMPORTANT NOTICE

The purpose of this book is to educate. While every effort has been made to ensure accuracy, it is not intended to replace any medical advice or to halt proper medical treatment. Rather, this book provides information for the reader to utilize as he or she sees fit as part of a personal health and wellness plan. This book is sold with the understanding that the author shall have no liability for any injury or harm alleged to be caused directly or indirectly by its contents.

Contents

Introduction

We live in a world where convenience outweighs nutrition. We have been conditioned to believe food must come in a box, can, or bag and be easy and quick to prepare. We eat processed and empty calories as the bulk of our diet because they are more convenient than making the effort to eat healthily. Moreover, we miss out on the experiences of socializing and interacting with our families as we cook and prepare meals. The result of this unhealthy diet is a significant increase in chronic illnesses and degenerative diseases. In fact, poor nutrition is a major contributing factor in the three leading causes of death among Americans: heart disease, cancer, and stroke. Contrary to logic, the diets consumed in industrialized nations are inferior when compared to those consumed decades ago. In the past, only the wealthy could afford the luxury of unhealthy meals. Ironically, so-called "unindustrialized" communities have lower levels of chronic illnesses and typically avoid the common diseases that are so prevalent in affluent societies. Poor nutritional habits slowly weaken our immune systems and breakdown our resistance to diseases. This may take years to become apparent, but poor nutritional habits will eventually result in negative consequences.

We have virtually as many opinions regarding healthy food choices as there are people in the world. So how do we determine what a health-promoting diet is? The intent of this book is to provide nutritional guidance and empower individuals to make correct dietary choices. Its guidance can benefit everyone regardless of race, religion, or socioeconomic status. It is based upon a revelation, essentially a guide to nutrition, as given from God to His prophet Joseph Smith. Even though it is a revelation directed toward members of The Church of Jesus Christ of

1

Latter-day Saints, it does not preclude people of all religious denominations from benefiting from its counsel. The information is offered for the benefit of all, and not by constraint or force. In other words, you can take the advice or leave it. It is my desire and obligation to share my knowledge of health and nutrition and to educate and inform you of appropriate dietary measures, then let you determine if these suggestions make sense for you and your family. I hope that all who read this book will gain knowledge beneficial to their health and the health of their families. Hopefully, the thoughts presented will establish daily dietary habits that promote the health of the body and the soul.

Unfortunately we tend to focus on a small portion of the Word of Wisdom: the don'ts. This is despite the fact that the bulk of this revelation teaches us what we *should* eat. In order to live the Word of Wisdom to its fullest, we must incorporate the dos as well as avoid the don'ts. If you follow the wise counsel the Lord has given, you will achieve optimal health and wellness. Of course, this doesn't mean you will be disease-free or illness-free, but you will establish the greatest possible health for you. Or in other words, become your best, healthy self. Moreover you may decrease your health care expenses in the process. An interesting article recently proclaimed that if no Americans were fat, the combined savings in health, food, clothing, and efficiencies would result in a savings of $4,270 per American, or $487 billion.[1] In the United States, more money is spent on health care than on education. If everyone followed the Lord's counsel, I am confident there would be less disease, less disability, and further enriched lives. We would live not just longer, but live healthier and have greater opportunity to share our lives to the fullest with those we love.

The counsel in this book is not meant to encourage extremism in diet but to promote thoughtful deliberation of one's current nutritional practices and state of health. Balance is key, and it takes effort, but it is not difficult to incorporate. Besides, isn't your health worth it?

Principles of this revelation and the suggestions contained in this book are best taught when children are young, but they can be incorporated at any age. The sooner a person learns proper nutritional habits, the earlier he or she can establish personal optimal health. My desire is that parents will learn better dietary habits from this book and teach them to their children, thus enabling them to perpetuate good habits to each subsequent generation, breaking the current trend toward convenience at the expense of nutrition. Ultimately I hope this will result in healthier generations and end the cycle of obesity, disease, and poor health currently being propagated by unhealthy dietary habits and lifestyle choices.

I possess a personal witness of the divinity and importance of this revelation. I have seen its benefits in my own life and the lives of others. President Gordon B. Hinckley said, "The code of health followed by the Latter-day Saints, which is so widely praised these days of cancer and heart research, is in reality a revelation given to Joseph Smith in 1833 as 'a word of wisdom' from the Lord (see D&C 89:1). In no conceivable way could it have come of the dietary literature of the time nor from the mind of the man who announced it. Today, in terms of medical research, it is a miracle whose observance has saved incalculable suffering and premature death for uncounted tens of thousands."[2] To his testimony I add mine, that the Word of Wisdom is a revelation from God, the observance of which will prevent unnecessary suffering and death and enhance the health of all who endeavor to live it to its fullest.

1

The Word *of* Wisdom

A Word of Wisdom, for the benefit of the council of high priests, assembled in Kirtland, and the church, and also the saints in Zion—To be sent greeting; not by commandment or constraint, but by revelation and the word of wisdom, showing forth the order and will of God in the temporal salvation of the saints in the last days—Given for a principle with promise, adapted to the capacity of the weak and the weakest of all saints, who are or can be called saints. Behold, verily, thus saith the Lord unto you: In consequence of evils and designs which do and will exist in the hearts of conspiring men in the last days, I have warned you, and forewarn you, by giving unto you this word of wisdom by revelation.

Doctrine & Covenants 89:1–4

Nutrition is an enormous and controversial subject. The information that can be found regarding this subject is vast, and the number of experts in nutrition is equally daunting. Numerous books purport to contain the best diet for your health when there is not one ideal diet, but many, based on the needs and circumstances of each person. We are all metabolically different, requiring different nutrients. Numerous fad diets claim to be the best for weight loss, but they all approach this matter in a different and often contradictory way. If you perform an Internet search for nutritional subjects, you will get an enormous number of people and websites all willing to share "expert" advice. Much of this advice is based on their desire to sell you a product or particular diet plan.

Eating healthy takes effort. But it is vital and plays the most critical role in our health. Nutrition truly is the foundation of your health. "You are what you eat" is more literal than some of us would like to believe. What we eat eventually enters and makes up the content of our blood stream. Our food is utilized as the building blocks of our body. Proper nourishment is necessary for cells to rebuild and function properly. Nutrition is particularly important for the growth and development of children and adolescents, but it remains important for all ages in order to reduce the risk of chronic illnesses. According to the American Institute for Cancer Research, 30 to 40 percent of cancers in 2008 were nutrition related.[1] If we altered our diet to include healthier and more nutritious choices, how many of the 553,888[2] cancer deaths per year could be avoided?

THE ROLE OF NUTRITION IN DISEASE

Many diseases and conditions are associated with poor nutrition, including cardiovascular disease, stroke, diabetes, osteoporosis, and obesity.[3] According to one study, about 16 percent of mortality in men and 9 percent in women could be eliminated by appropriate nutritional behaviors.[4] This is a conservative number, in my opinion. I believe that *most* disease results from poor nutrition, which provides the perfect environment for disease to flourish. Many foreign and disease-causing microbes will only thrive and cause illness if given the right environment and a host with a weak immune system. How many deaths could be avoided with a few small changes in dietary habits? A significant number. Not to mention the improved quality of life that would be achieved. Yes, Americans are living longer than ever, but what quality of life are we enjoying? Quantity does not always equal quality! We are not living healthier, better-quality lives. This is obvious as we see our nursing homes full of sick, decrepit, and crippled elderly. We accept certain illnesses and conditions as a normal part of aging, when this is not true. Many of these conditions and illnesses are present because of poor dietary and lifestyle choices.

Some would say that it is too expensive to eat healthy meals. In the short term, it certainly is more expensive to purchase healthy products instead of products devoid of proper and essential nutrients. But can you really put a price tag on your health? How much is your good health worth? In the long term, healthy eating and providing your body proper nutrition will save you untold dollars in health care costs and lost wages. The authors of *The China Study* state that "eating the right way would largely obviate the enormous costs of using drugs, as well as their side effects. Fewer people would need to wage lengthy, expensive battles with chronic disease in hospitals over their last years of life. Health care costs would drop and medical mistakes would wane as premature death plummeted. In essence, our health care system would finally protect and promote our health as it is meant to do."[5] You can pay a little more now to eat healthy or pay a lot later in health care expenses. Another question may be the genetics factor. This is, of course, a factor that must be considered in disease, but much like a light switch has the capability to provide light, it cannot do so without an external factor; our bodies may have the genetic predisposition to a disease or condition but will not manifest this condition unless an internal switch is turned on. This internal switch is often nutrition. The more substandard our nutrition, the greater the possibility of turning switches on. A gardener will tell you that a seed is no good unless you can provide the proper soil, nutrients, water, and sunlight required for that seed to mature and develop into a plant. Theoretically, if we were to keep our body healthy enough, we would not allow the disease (seed) the proper nutrients and environment (soil) to develop. Proper dietary habits provide proper nutrients for optimal functioning of the immune system and a less hospitable environment for disease to develop.

Nutrition plays a crucial role in our immune system. The immune system is a complex system of specialized cells and organs that work together to prevent invasion by foreign substances and to remove foreign and harmful invaders if they do invade the body. There are two classes of specialized cells, called lymphocytes, in the body: B cells, which circulate in the blood locating and marking antigens (foreign invaders) for destruction; and T cells, which patrol for invaders but also play a role in the removal and destruction of antigens. Poor nutrition primarily affects the alarm portion of the immune system, which notifies the body of foreign invaders and marks them for destruction. This allows these antigens to progress freely through the body undetected. This is similar to having an alarm on your home without any power supplied to the alarm unit. Eventually disease or illness will result. Nutrient deficiencies can also suppress the immune system. This suppression allows the invaders more activity and opportunity to cause damage, disease, or illness. Proper nutrition is the body's best defense against foreign invaders by supporting optimal immune system function.

Obesity is an epidemic in the United States, mostly caused by poor dietary and lifestyle behaviors. The more extra weight an individual carries, the greater the risk for chronic diseases. Being overweight increases your risk of diabetes, arthritis, osteoarthritis, high blood pressure, and cardiovascular disease. Obesity can also be emotionally taxing, as it devastates a person's self-esteem and confidence. This lack of confidence in physical appearance may drive the obese person to avoid social situations and interactions with others. Thus he or she may inadvertently shut out the help and assistance needed to begin the path to better health.

A new miracle weight-loss pill, surgery, or plan is suggested every day, it seems. Surgeons modify the stomach, making it as small as a thumb; others promote harmful drugs; and still others encourage dangerous diet or lifestyle choices, all in the name of losing weight. Unscrupulous people take the money of overweight and obese persons, providing little more than false hope that their miracle "cure" will result in weight loss. Innumerable weight-loss programs and diets exist, some backed by doctors or other nutrition experts. Some diets advocate high-protein, low-carbohydrate diets, when in fact a high-carbohydrate diet is the healthiest you can consume. The important factor is the type of carbohydrates you consume. Refined sugar and white flour are aptly called "empty calories" because they supply lots of calories but few essential nutrients and will cause weight gain. The bottom line is that a healthy and proper diet combined with moderate exercise is the best way to maintain a healthy weight. We simply can't continue to sit in front of the television for hours snacking on junk food and expect to maintain a healthy weight.

Chronic illnesses and degenerative diseases are no longer plagues that only affect the elderly. More and more, our children and very young adults are succumbing to life-altering and crippling illnesses. Diseases that used to be considered adult diseases are more common among children, including high blood pressure, asthma, and diabetes. All of these diseases can cause limitations on the activities of these children, resulting in an inferior quality of life. The incidence of childhood asthma has increased approximately 247 percent in the last twenty-five years.[6] Two studies concluded that type 1 diabetes (a chronic condition in which the pancreas does not produce enough insulin to properly control blood sugar) has not only increased significantly but also strikes children at a younger age.[7,8] It is tragic to watch children suffer through such horrible and debilitating diseases, and parents need to make a more concerted effort to provide proper nutrition to their children, which enables them the best chance to avoid such diseases.

CAN STUDIES AND EXPERTS BE TRUSTED?

If you ask five nutritionists for an opinion on a particular nutrient, you are likely to receive five different views. Often, studies and scientific publications regarding the same nutrient contradict each other. Look at the butter versus margarine debate for an example. One study will assert that margarine is healthier, while another asserts butter is better, with both sides of the debate presenting "scientific" data to back up their claims. Who can you believe when contradictory studies exist?

These studies are often biased depending on who is funding the study. For example, one study funded by the corporate parent of Lipton tea suggests that up to forty ounces of unsweetened coffee or tea and twelve ounces of beer daily is healthy.[9] This study asserted that unsweetened tea and coffee are acceptable substitutes for water. It is quite comical to believe that a study funded and initiated by Lipton would produce any other results. Those that conducted the study had a vested interest in ascertaining this conclusion.

Data may be interpreted favorably or unfavorably based on the views and or beliefs of the individual conducting the study. If a scientist has a particular view about a nutrient, it is human nature to hope for favorable results for that nutrient. The scientist will do everything possible to prove his or her hypothesis or belief. It is the equivalent of Ford Motor Company requesting and paying for a study to determine if their vehicles are reliable. Bias frequently sneaks into studies and articles, probably more than we know. In fact, an article published in *PLoS Medicine*, a peer-reviewed journal, concluded that food industry funding of nutrition-related scientific articles may bias the articles in preference to the sponsor's products, with substantial implications for public health.[10] This article found that 87 percent of studies funded by an industry had results favorable or neutral to the industry, while only 61 percent of non-industry-funded studies were favorable or neutral to the industry. This is a significant difference and demonstrates the bias inherent to industry-funded studies. Studies are often designed to ensure a specific outcome and results are frequently manipulated and interpreted sympathetically toward the sponsor, or the desired outcome of the individual conducting the study. When a new study is released, touting a benefit or consequence of a product, it would be prudent to investigate the funding of the study and the background of the person or persons who conducted the study.

WHERE TO FIND UNFAILING HEALTH AND NUTRITION GUIDANCE

With this much information to sort through and with contradictory scientific studies commonplace, are we then doomed to never have accurate and unbiased information about nutrition? The answer to that question is no. Is there a better source than God when it comes to nutrition? He is the designer and creator of our bodies and knows what is best for them. He is the master nutritionist, chemist, and biologist. In contrast to the philosophies of men and the scientific community, God remains constant and unchanging. He wants His children to be healthy and has given us a blueprint of what constitutes proper and healthful nutrition in the Word of Wisdom. Given the complexity of the human organism, who better to consult about nutrition than our Creator?

He will not force the Word of Wisdom on any of His children, but it is His will that we are healthy and have the knowledge available to take care of our bodies. God has offered us some of His wisdom and knowledge of nutrition and the human body, and we may choose to accept or reject that information. Not only does He offer us this knowledge, but He provides us a promise that we will have optimal health, both physically and mentally, if we follow His counsel contained in the Word of Wisdom. He has made it simple and manageable to follow so that all may reap the benefits of His wisdom and knowledge.

You don't have to be a genius to follow His code of health; you only need knowledge and the desire to do so.

CONSPIRING MEN AND COMPANIES
SEEK TO DESTROY YOUR HEATLH

We live in a time where profit and wealth are considered over health and wellness—a time where many "conspiring men" produce and sell products that adversely affect health, despite having full knowledge that these products are unhealthy. Selfish and greedy men pad their wallets at the detriment of those who consume their products. Misleading and fraudulent advertisements are created by cunning men in order to create desirability for their products. The consequence of this is poor health. An example of this is a study published in the *Annals of Internal Medicine*, which indicates the need for long-term use of smoking cessation products—despite the fact these same products are known to have side effects such as suicidal thoughts, seizures, and loss of consciousness. The four experts that conducted the research were funded by the manufacturers of smoking cessation products that had billions of dollars to gain by getting such a report published.[11] This appears to be nothing more than telling the pharmaceutical companies what they want to hear in order to generate billions of more dollars in profits. Even Harvard Medical School has recently indicated they feel the influence of pharmaceutical companies is rampant in their schools because of the millions of dollars these companies pour into this educational institution.

Conspiring men are not new. Benefiting from conspiracy was had among our earliest ancestors. As noted in the Bible, Cain killed his brother, Abel, for gain. The father of all lies used man's appetite for greed against Cain, and Cain paid dearly for it (Genesis 4:8–16). Satan continues his desire and purpose of creating misery for man today. He uses the same desire for gain and "conspiring men" as his pawns in his wicked game to inflict disease, sickness, pain, misery, and death upon man. Ultimately Satan's goal is to separate man from God. His methods are subtle and often difficult to detect.

The cigarette industry is an appropriate example of "conspiring men." It concealed and obscured evidence that cigarettes were unhealthy and had been implicated in many chronic illnesses. Phillip Morris, the largest cigarette manufacturer in the world, knew at least by the 1980s that secondhand smoke was extremely toxic but hid this truth for decades.[12] The company covered up this information because they did not want their product to be adversely affected. There was no thought for human health, only thought for protection of profit. They did not want to lose their gain, despite the destruction it was proliferating among men. The only reason for a product such as cigarettes to exist is to provide profit to government agencies through taxes and the cigarette manufacturers. Why else would a product linked to cancer, heart disease, stroke, emphysema, and premature death be allowed to continue on the market? The government has pulled other products for lesser offenses than this, but continues to turn a blind eye toward the cigarette industry.

Other harmful substances have been portrayed as socially acceptable by various means. Television and movies are full of instances where drugs and alcohol are portrayed as customary. People try to justify the use of drugs for medicinal purposes when better alternatives are clearly available. Advertising and marketing campaigns bombard us with promotions to represent alcohol, smoking, and other harmful products as normal and popular. It is imperative that we stand firm in avoiding harmful substances and not yield to these addicting and health-deteriorating products. If we stand firm, we will be able to avoid the trap of being addicted to harmful products. Some products are so powerful that trying them once can initiate a biological craving for the product. After continued use this creates a physical addiction almost impossible for some to overcome. The addicted person becomes hopeless and forlorn with little hope of conquering such a gripping addiction.

How often have we seen businesses collapse because of the unsavory actions of managers, executives, and owners? Some companies failed during the financial crisis of 2008 because unscrupulous executives manipulated their companies' accounting books so they could receive their bonuses. In an effort to keep up with the Joneses, people cheat, embezzle, lie, and steal. Moral decency, honesty, and integrity have been replaced by greed, power, and wealth. Man's desire for profit that existed in the time of Adam continues in full force today. The term *conspiring men* is applicable to more than just the manufacturers of addictive drugs and products. This term could easily be applied to any person who willingly sells a harmful product for gain. The fast-food industry is a good example of conspiring men that is not often thought of. They continue to advertise and market their products despite established adverse side effects. They sell products that are full of calories, fat, sugar, and salt, which contribute to the poor health of Americans. In today's age of instant information, do they really expect us to believe they don't know the food they sell contributes to negative health consequences? Absolutely not. They know about the detrimental affects of the food they sell but choose to ignore them for the sake of profits.

THE WORD OF WISDOM IS YOUR
BODY'S OWNER'S MANUAL

With these circumstances is it any wonder that God sent the Word of Wisdom by greeting and not by commandment? If He had sent it by commandment at the time the revelation was revealed, countless people would have come under immediate condemnation because of their addictions. Instead, the Lord provided a period of time for His saints to familiarize themselves with the revelation and relinquish problematic addictions. He, in His usual loving and kind way, sent the Word of Wisdom to give us counsel, guidance, and direction, while still giving us time to overcome addictions to unhealthful products and habits. After sufficient time had passed, Church President Brigham Young announced that the revelation was a command of the Lord,[13] and members of the Church were now expected to live by its precepts.

We are told that our body is a temple (1 Corinthians 3:16). Should we not then treat our body as we would treat the temple of God? How many of us would bring toxic and poisonous substances into the temple with the full knowledge that they would harm the temple? We need to take care of our bodies and respect the creation of our Maker by listening to and obeying His counsel. Many of us take better care of our vehicles than we do our bodies. If a vehicle manufacturer recommends oil changes at regular intervals (which all of them do), we take our vehicle to be serviced at regular intervals. We rely upon the owner's manual to tell us how to best take care of our vehicles, yet we disregard the manual the Lord has provided for our body. What a tragedy that we have our owner's manual in front of us yet choose to leave it on the shelf, ignoring the instructions contained therein. If this same practice were applied to our vehicles, they would quickly deteriorate and fail. This is the same path that those who choose to ignore the Word of Wisdom are following. Our bodies requires proper care and nourishment to function optimally, and they will deteriorate and break down if we continue to neglect them.

2

Healthy *and* Unhealthy Beverages

That inasmuch as any man drinketh wine or strong drink among you, behold it is not good, neither meet in the sight of your Father, only in assembling yourselves together to offer up your sacraments before him.

And, behold, this should be wine, yea, pure wine of the grape of the vine, of your own make.

And again strong drinks are not for the belly, but for the washing of your bodies. And again, hot drinks are not for the body or the belly.

Doctrine & Covenants 89:5–7, 9

Families are torn apart and lives are lost from the abuse of alcohol. Alcohol is a drug, a central nervous system depressant, and a poison that harms the organs. It suppresses inhibitions and moral sense and therefore appropriate self-control. Character is weakened and immoral acts are more likely when under its influence. Even small amounts of alcohol can change behavior, generally making the consumer more careless and irresponsible. Many people do things under the influence of alcohol that they would not normally do. Alcohol gives us a false sense of well-being while decreasing motor skills, decreasing muscle control, reducing coordination, impairing judgment, and retarding ability to reason. This is why people under the influence of alcohol drive so erratically and have slurred speech.

Unfortunately the actions of those who choose to drive while impaired with alcohol or other substances greatly affect the lives of others every day. Not only do they ruin their own health and lives, but they also ruin the lives of others. Alcohol consumption is the third leading preventable cause of death in the United States.[1] Every day, more than 207 deaths are attributed to this destructive drug.[2] Alcohol can often lead to behavioral changes such as anger and violence. Just ask the children or spouse of an angry drunk. The home of a drunk is no place for children. Often children in this situation will seek solace at the house of a friend to avoid the negative interaction of their father or mother. The Lord knows the negative consequences of drinking alcohol and strong drinks and therefore warns us not to partake of them.

THE ADDICTIVE POWER OF ALCOHOL

Alcohol is an addictive drug. Many people are slaves to this addiction, and both they and their families suffer because of it. Numerous beneficial programs exist to help overcome this addiction, including a program instituted by The Church of Jesus Christ of Latter-day Saints. However, it is so much better to avoid alcohol completely, thus avoiding the addiction altogether.

The costs of alcohol addiction are enormous—financially, physically, and emotionally—to individuals, families, and communities. Some are so addicted to alcohol they seek a temporary buzz from the content of odd sources such as extracts that contain alcohol, cough syrup, and even rubbing alcohol. Commonly this method is used by those not of legal age to consume alcohol, such as teenagers. This destructive routine only leads a person down a more devastating path as they try to satisfy their addiction.

THE NEGATIVE EFFECTS OF
ALCOHOL ON YOUR HEALTH

There are many negative effects of alcohol consumption on your health. Because alcohol is a diuretic, it causes rapid water loss, leaching water from the body. It depletes vitamins and minerals from your body, particularly magnesium, folic acid, vitamin B12, thiamine, pyridoxine (vitamin B6), vitamin A, and zinc, which all play critical roles in the processes and function of the body. Excessive alcohol consumption can lead to deficiencies in these key nutrients and a range of disease related to their deficiency, and can lead to liver cirrhosis, various cancers, and unintentional injuries. Alcohol irritates the intestines and the liver, the primary organ of detoxification. The liver attempts to detoxify alcohol from the body, but when it gets overwhelmed, liver cells may be destroyed or damaged leading to fat deposits in the liver, liver inflammation, or permanent scarring (cirrhosis). The liver acts as a filter, removing wastes, poisons, toxins, and excess hormones. Since the liver is the foundation of the body's detoxification system, body toxicity can result if the liver is damaged.

IS MODERATE CONSUMPTION OF ALCOHOL
A HEALTHY PRACTICE?

Much information has been published about the health benefits of moderate wine consumption, especially red wine. Some health professionals recommend moderate consumption of alcohol—one drink per day for women and two for men—as a healthful practice. These assertions have some truth and scientific basis. Some studies have in fact found that moderate alcohol consumption reduces the risk of heart disease and cancer.[3, 4, 5] However, the studies and especially the wine industry fail to inform that grape juice offers similar benefits as red wine. In addition, alcohol studies are contradictory with one claiming health benefits such as reduced risk of heart disease,[6] while others suggest alcohol doubles the risk of breast cancer,[7] increases the risk of small intestinal bacterial overgrowth,[8] and cognitive decline in those over age 65.[9] Who should you believe? The Lord has provided the definitive answer. Wine and alcohol should not be consumed.

The benefits that are derived from wine consumption are a result of the phytochemicals, antioxidants, and polyphenols contained in grapes, particularly in the skin of grapes. In fact, the concentration of the flavonoid polyphenol resveratrol is much higher in a serving of grapes (including the grape skins) than it is in wine itself. Red wine contains from 1.5 to 3.0 milligrams of resveratrol per liter, while fresh grape skins contain 5 to 10 milligrams per serving.[10]

THE POWER OF ANTIOXIDANTS TO COMBAT
FREE RADICAL DAMAGE

To better understand what antioxidants do in the body, one must understand free radicals. Free radicals are molecules produced during the normal energy-producing processes within our cells. Free radicals may originate from metabolism, inflammation, stress, and exposure to toxic chemicals. In fact, your body's immune system uses free radicals in the process of destroying foreign bodies such as viruses and bacteria. The same process that damages healthy cells also damages bacteria and viruses. Molecules normally contain paired electrons. When molecules are missing an electron, they become free radicals, and thus try to capture an electron from a healthy molecule. When they take an electron from a healthy molecule, they damage it and the DNA contained therein. When the molecules of a cell become damaged, its DNA is damaged, and it then mutates, growing and reproducing abnormally and rapidly. Think of it this way: if you attempted to make a copy from a document covered in water and mud, the resultant copy would not resemble the original document very closely. Then if you continued to make copies of the subsequent copy, you would experience further degradation of the document's quality. The end result of damaged DNA and cells is illness and disease.

Antioxidants prevent damage to cells within your body. Oxygen is critical to life but plays a damaging role as well, called oxidation. Some examples of oxidation are the rusting that takes place when metal is left exposed to the elements, or the browning that occurs to apple and banana slices when left exposed to oxygen. Oxidation can have a negative effect on the body as well, and if left unchecked, it eventually damages cells and inhibits proper functioning. This malfunction can then lead to cancer, heart disease, diabetes, and a host of other conditions. Antioxidants work in a chemical process and through exchange of electrons to neutralize oxidation, but this process is only effective when there is an adequate supply and continual renewal of the antioxidants. In the effort to combat the oxidation process, antioxidants are oxidized and require replenishment by another antioxidant to continue the battle. It's kind of like sending in the cavalry when you see your front lines need extra support. The body's need for antioxidants depends on its current condition. For example, someone with arthritis or another chronic illness will have greater requirements for antioxidants than someone who does not.

Flavonoids are complex chemicals contained within plants, especially fruits, vegetables, and whole grains. They act as powerful antioxidants within the body, assisting in the battle against free radicals. Some scientists and doctors believe that flavonoids may hold the key to controlling cancer, both as a preventative and as a treatment.[11] Grapes contain the flavonoid resveratrol, which is an outstanding antioxidant and has the ability to lower LDL (bad cholesterol), and reduce the risk of heart disease.[12, 13, 14] Other important phytochemicals found in grapes that work in the battle against free radicals are proanthocyanidins, saponins, and anthocyanins.

Alcohol has been implicated as a contributing factor in heart disease, high blood pressure, heart failure, and stroke. Drinking too much of it can raise triglyceride (fats in the blood) levels.[15] High triglyceride levels are associated with greater risk of heart disease. Alcohol is not meant for internal consumption but rather for external use. It is best to keep alcohol to its intended use as an antiseptic "for the washing of your bodies" (Doctrine and Covenants 89:7) In this function it inhibits growth of many microorganisms, including viruses, bacteria, and fungi.

STRONG DRINKS: TEA AND COFFEE

We have been told that the phrase "strong drinks" indicates coffee and tea. Joseph Smith, as quoted by Joel H. Johnson, stated, "[Tea and coffee] are what the Lord meant when he said 'hot drinks.'"[16] This is also a logical assumption, because the common "hot drinks" of Joseph Smith's time were coffee and tea. Brigham Young spoke of this when he said "I have heard it argued that tea and coffee are not mentioned [in the Word of Wisdom]; that is very true; but what were the people in the habit of taking as hot drinks when the revelation was given? Tea and coffee. We were not in the habit of drinking water very hot, but tea and coffee—the beverages in common use."[17] In addition, Victor Ludlow asserts "The Word of Wisdom counsels against drinking 'hot drinks,' which have been identified by early Church leaders as coffee and tea. 'Tea' refers to the standard tea derived from the tea plant, sometimes called black or green tea. The Word of Wisdom has not been interpreted as proscribing herbal teas, stating that 'all wholesome herbs God hath ordained for the constitution, nature, and use of man (D&C 89:10)."[18] Because statements have been made that tea is against the Word of Wisdom, we have made tea a negative word in LDS culture. We do not differentiate between beneficial herbal teas and standard teas, simply stating that all tea is against the Word of Wisdom. Why, if God has stated that herbs are beneficial for man, would we assume that they are not beneficial when consumed in tea form? This goes against all logic and reason. Technically any plant having leaves that are boiled in water to create a beverage could be considered a tea. Does this mean if you boil carrot leaves and drink the water you are breaking the Word of Wisdom?

IS CAFFEINE THE REASON TEA AND COFFEE ARE AGAINST THE WORD OF WISDOM?

While all coffee (yes even decaffeinated) and some teas contain the drug caffeine, many other substances are concerning in these common beverages, namely the xanthine alkaloids theophylline and theobromine and the tannins they contains: fluoride, chlorogenic acid, and oxalate.

Given the popularity of Mitt Romney's run for president in 2012, much ado has been made about the Church's stance on caffeine. Because this issue has become such a contentious and confusing topic among members of the Church, the Church issued an official statement of clarification. It reads, *"Despite what was reported, the Church revelation spelling out health practices (Doctrine and Covenants 89) does not mention the use of caffeine. The Church's health guidelines prohibits alcoholic drinks, smoking or chewing of tobacco, and "hot drinks" — taught by Church leaders to refer specifically to tea and coffee."*

Although the Word of Wisdom does not specifically forbid caffeine, Bishop H. Burke Peterson had the following to say about it: "We should notice the word *wholesome* and always consider the things that we take into our body as to whether they are wholesome or not. The scripture continues 'All these to be used with prudence and thanksgiving'

(D&C 89:11). . . . We know that cola drinks contain the drug caffeine. We know that caffeine is not wholesome nor prudent for the use of our bodies. It is only sound judgment to conclude that cola drinks and others that contain caffeine or other harmful ingredients should not be used."[19] Drinks that contain harmful and habit-forming drugs should therefore be avoided. It is important for everyone to prayerfully consider what this means for them, as the Lord will not command in all things. He leaves us room to make our own decisions and choices, and will not force anyone to live healthily.

THE DANGERS OF CAFFEINE

Caffeine is the most abused behavior-modifying drug in the world. In excessive amounts, caffeine is addictive, causes jumpiness and heart palpitations, reduces mental function, can restrict liver function, reduces fertility in women, causes headaches in some people, leaches B vitamins from the body, and depletes essential minerals (especially calcium) from the body.[20] When caffeine first enters the blood stream, it is very stimulating, but after its immediate effects wear off, it actually depresses the system causing a crash in your energy levels. This up-and-down effect deceives the user to believe he or she feels better when under the influence of caffeine. It provides a false sense of more energy and liveliness. Because caffeine is a stimulant, it may cause insomnia as well as hyperactivity. The list of negative effects of caffeine continues with osteoporosis, diarrhea, increased blood pressure, increased cholesterol and triglyceride levels, fibrocystic breast disease, birth defects and mis-carriages, kidney stones, increased incidence of some cancers, prostate enlargement, adrenal exhaustion, increased heartburn, and anxiety.[21] Why anyone would want to consume large quantities of a drink that contains such a destructive drug each day is unfathomable. Is it any wonder Americans are plagued with health problems when we drink caffeinated soda, coffee, and teas as water substitutes? I know many people who feel they could not make it through the day without indulging in these unhealthy beverages. They have to make trip after trip to the pop or coffee machine to maintain the feeling of energy they lose when not consuming caffeinated beverages. Their bodies have become used to having these stimulants and in many ways now require them. The brain receives craving signals from the body for these substances because of their addictive nature. A word of caution for those who want to quit caffeinated beverages. It is wise to slowly wean yourself from these addictive substances, because quitting abruptly can cause severe withdrawal symptoms, including headache, irritability, muscle aches, and constipation. It is best to gradually decrease your intake of these beverages over an extended period of time.

In addition, the sugary syrup contained in soda creates more desire to consume them freely, making them in some ways worse than coffee and tea that are consumed slowly because of their bitter flavor. Both diet and regular soda are significant contributing factors to the obesity epidemic.[22] Quite simply, soda should rarely be consumed except as an occasional treat.

Energy drinks have become very popular recently. Unfortunately, these drinks provide energy by injecting significant quantities of caffeine and/or other stimulants into the bloodstream. These drinks are targeted to teens, despite a warning label on some of them that indicates they should not be consumed by anyone under age eighteen. One energy drink even boasts three hundred milligrams of caffeine in one 8.4-ounce serving. Sadly caffeinism, or an overdose of caffeine, can occur with as little as 250 milligrams in those who are genetically susceptible. The FDA limits the amount of caffeine contained in food products to seventy-one milligrams per

Product	Caffeine (mg)
Coffee (6 oz. cup)	
Drip	*175*
Percolated	*132*
Instant regular	*62*
Decaffeinated	*2*
Tea	
Black	*47*
Green	*30–50*
White	*15*
Soft Drinks (12 oz. can)	
Mountain Dew	*54*
Dr Pepper	*47*
Pepsi	*38*
Diet Coke	*47*
Energy Drinks	
Full Throttle (16 oz.)	*144*
Monster (16 oz.)	*160*
Candy Bars	
Hershey Bar (1.55 oz)	*9*

Resource: USDA National Nutrient Database for Standard Reference, 2007.

twelve ounces. However, energy drinks are labeled as dietary supplements, so they don't fall under these restrictions. Energy drink manufacturers go unchecked, loading their products with as much of this addictive substance as possible, thus creating the desire to consume more and more of the product. Five hundred to six hundred milligrams of caffeine can cause anxiety, muscle tremors, and abnormal heart rhythms. Recently, many people have succumbed to the caffeine content of these energy drinks and been hospitalized. Some have even died due to caffeine overdose. Even athletes in superb shape are not immune to an overdose of caffeine.

WHY TEA IS HARMFUL TO YOUR HEALTH

Black, green, and white teas originate from the same tea plant (*Camellia sinensis*). They differ in the manner they are processed. Black tea is processed further than green tea. Green tea is partially fermented—the oxidation of the plant polyphenols in the tea leaf—whereas black tea is fully fermented. White tea leaves are harvested at a younger age than both black and green tea products and are not fermented at all. Green tea has received rave press regarding its antioxidant properties, which indeed it contains. It is also touted as a weight-loss miracle because of its ability to induce thermogenesis and boost metabolism. Green tea contains powerful antioxidant compounds that have therapeutic value as natural medicines. However, looking only at green tea's antioxidant properties dismisses the hundreds of other biochemical compounds it contains and their possible health benefits and risks. The tea plant contains the xanthine alkaloids caffeine, theobromine, and theophylline, all of which are central nervous system stimulants and diuretics. The tea plant also contains significant amounts of fluoride, tannin, and some oxalate. Dr. Clifford Stratton states, "The xanthines stimulate the brain and spinal cord, increase heart action, constrict blood vessels feeding the brain (that's why extra-strength aspirin compounds help a headache so dramatically), relieve respiratory distress by relaxing certain muscles, strengthen the contractions of arm and leg muscles, increase the production of urine, increase the amount of acid secreted into the stomach, and generally increase body metabolism."[23] Too many xanthines in the system my cause diarrhea, dizziness, trembling, frequent urination, and insomnia. There are some people who believe it is okay to drink iced tea because it is not a "hot drink." However, they are incorrect in this thinking because iced tea is often derived from the *Camellia sinensis* plant and carries the same health risks. Just because it is not hot does not mean it is not prohibited by the Word of Wisdom. All drinks that are injurious or addictive should be avoided. Moreover, even drinks that are too hot can damage the mouth, tongue, and esophagus and should be consumed with great caution.

Excessive tea consumption stimulates overproduction of gastric acid and may lead to indigestion. In addition, drinking too much tea may lead to kidney stones because of its oxalate content. The stimulants in the tea plant may also overstimulate the kidneys, causing permanent damage. It appears theobromine is more irritating to the kidneys than caffeine. Excessive tea consumption has been linked with aggravating premenstrual symptoms[24] and may lead to incontinence and frequent or urgent impulse to urinate.[25]

Theobromine is suspected of being toxic to the endocrine system (the body system comprising organs and glands that secrete hormones to control normal physiological processes), toxic to the liver and gastrointestinal tract, a neurotoxin (substances that cause adverse affects on the central nervous system), and implicated as a contributing factor in adverse effects to the reproductive system.[26] Because of its diuretic nature, theobromine also increases the body's requirement for fluid.

Theophylline's negative effects are similar to those of caffeine, but it is considered slightly more toxic. It stimulates the heart and respiratory system. Because it is a bronchodilator, it is sometimes used medicinally in the treatment of asthma. Theophylline may cause irritability, nausea, or headaches. Combined, theobromine, caffeine, and theophylline strengthen their diuretic and stimulant properties. The power and strength of this combination can result in more frequent and serious adverse side effects.

The chlorogenic acid content in coffee and black tea increases plasma homocystiene levels, a predictive factor for cardiovascular disease.[27] This suggests that the more coffee and black tea consumed, the greater the risk of heart disease. Americans could have a significant reduction in the risk of heart disease by eliminating these two harmful drinks that are so frequently consumed.

Some people switch from coffee to tea, believing it to be a healthier beverage. Unfortunately, the adverse effects of tea from the *Camellia sinensis* plant are similar to those of coffee. The *Camellia sinensis* plant contains high amounts of naturally occurring fluoride, derived from air and soil pollution. The Environmental Protection Agency has set the drinking standard for fluoride at four milligrams per liter and a secondary standard of two milligrams per liter to protect against dental fluorosis,[28] a condition caused by excessive intake of fluoride, resulting in mottling of the teeth. One liter of green or black tea contains anywhere from 1.0mg to 1.9mg of fluoride alone. The average bottle of green tea is approximately one-half liter, and one eight-ounce cup of black tea is equivalent to almost one-quarter liter. These figures indicate that many people are drinking enough tea to consume an unhealthy amount of fluoride every day. This is also assuming that the water they use to make the tea is not fluoridated. If the water is fluoridated, the level of fluoride increases dramatically, as does the toxicity of the tea. Astonishingly, fluoride is more poisonous than lead. In excessive amounts, it has been linked to cancer, Alzheimer's disease, poor brain development in children, decreased thyroid activity, increased risk of bone fractures, atherosclerosis, dental fluorosis, and nervous system problems.[29]

Tannins are defensive chemicals found in plants to deter predators from consuming the plant. The same substance that gives tea its bitter flavor wards off animals and insects that may otherwise consume it. Coffee contains smaller quantities of tannic acid than tea. The tannin content in tea increases according to the age of the leaf. The older the leaf, the more tannin it contains. Approximately 7 to 14 percent of tea leaf composition is tannins. Research has shown a correlation between tannins and cancer of the esophagus.[30] Tannic acid can also cause indigestion and stomach ulcers.

THE HAZARDS OF COFFEE

Millions of people start their day with a cup of coffee. They continue drinking this beverage throughout the day, cup after cup. The caffeine content in coffee makes it a significant contributor to caffeine abuse. This is such a common beverage and practice that many see the LDS Church's restriction of coffee as odd. Coffee is such a strong drink that it often creates chemical dependence. Physical symptoms of withdrawal, including headache, difficulty concentrating, and fatigue, are common when the usual dose of coffee is reduced. The same three xanthine alkaloids (theobromine, theophylline, and caffeine) in tea are contained in coffee, so the same effects are expected. One big difference is that coffee contains significantly more caffeine than tea—depending on the coffee, almost four times more than black tea, and more than five times the amount in green tea (see table on page) According to Dr. Kaslow, the following are health issues associated with coffee and caffeine: exhausted adrenal glands (the stimulating effect of caffeine causes the adrenals to secrete the hormone adrenaline, the overuse of which exhausts them); severe blood sugar swings; acid imbalance (coffee stimulates the excess secretion of acid in the stomach, optimal health calls for an alkaline pH balance to the body); and essential mineral depletion (coffee causes the excretion of some minerals in the urine and inhibits the absorption of others).[31] One of the minerals that coffee reduces the absorption of is non-heme (iron from plant sources) iron, which increases the risk of anemia. The regular consumption of coffee may lead to cardiac sensitivity, abnormal heartbeats, anxiety, irritability, intestinal irritation, and insomnia.[32]

Some choose to drink decaffeinated coffee. However, the chemicals used to decaffeinate coffee create additional health concerns, particularly the large amounts of hydrogen peroxide. Frankly, there just isn't a healthful type of coffee to drink.

HEALTHY BEVERAGES YOU SHOULD CONSUME

When it comes to healthy beverages, water reigns supreme. Nothing quenches thirst as well as water. Purified drinking water is even better because it eliminates many of the heavy metals, microorganisms, and chemicals that are unfortunately contained in drinking water. A good starting point for water consumption is to drink six to eight eight-ounce glasses of water per day. To personalize your water consumption, drink half your body weight in ounces every day. For example, a 150-pound person would drink 75 ounces of water per day. Don't wait until you're thirsty to drink water. When your body has insufficient water, it sends this thirst signal so that you will drink the water it needs. This can be difficult in our busy and distracting lives, but is critical to our health. I find it easy to consume enough water by keeping a bottle of water at my desk, drinking it throughout the day. Water is fundamental to life as the primary component of all bodily fluids, including blood, lymph, tears, urine, sweat, and digestive juices. Water is essential to remove waste products of metabolism. In addition, water is involved in almost every bodily function, including most chemical reactions and the many life processes that take place in water. Our cells rely upon sufficient water to function properly.

Other healthy beverages are fruit and vegetable juices. But be careful of commercial juices that are full of added sugar. Juicing your own fresh fruit and vegetables is by far the healthiest and best method. This allows you to know exactly what is in your juice and control how much sugar is added, if any. Fruits are naturally high in sugar and most will taste sweet without the addition of refined sugar. Add apples or other sweet fruits to your vegetables to make them sweeter and more palatable. Juicing releases numerous health-promoting phytochemicals, including flavonoids beneficial for your health. When you make your own juice, you preserve good quantities of vitamins and some minerals. If you don't want to invest in a juicer or don't think you have the time, look for unsweetened juice at a health food store.

3

The Harmful Effects of Tobacco

And again, tobacco is not for the body, neither for the belly, and is not good for man, but is an herb for bruises and all sick cattle, to be used with judgment and skill.

Doctrine and Covenants 89:8

Ironically, the government works vigorously to protect us from air pollution while turning a blind eye to toxic and dangerous tobacco products. This fact is astonishing and another indication of the evil designs of conspiring men. Tobacco smoke contains more than four thousand chemicals,[1] of which eighty-one, so far, have been identified as carcinogenic.[2] Each puff of tobacco smoke inhaled wreaks havoc within the body as the body tries to detoxify an overabundance of unhealthy and toxic chemicals.

Most historians credit the Native Americans for instituting the use of tobacco for smoking. Christopher Columbus observed the Indians in this practice when he came to the Americas. In the mid-1900s, smoking was portrayed as being glamorous by movie stars, athletes, and political figures. All the while, the cigarette companies were producing massive quantities of a toxic product and earning significant profits at the expense of the smokers' health. Large sums of money were spent advertising cigarettes as sophisticated and prestigious, even healthful (for their appetite-suppressing effect), and unfortunately some of this advertising appeared to be geared toward teenagers and children. Many can remember the cartoon character Joe Camel that was used to market cigarettes. This was an obvious ploy to interest the young in this deplorable habit. These marketing programs, as well as the suppression of the scientific research implicating cigarettes in the cause of disease, were successful. It didn't take long for tobacco companies to secure a sizeable, addicted population to sell their products to.

THE HARMFUL EFFECTS OF SMOKING

Cigarette smoking is the most preventable cause of premature death and a major single cause of cancer mortality in the United States. In fact, cigarette smoking accounts for at least 30 percent of all cancer deaths and 87 percent of lung cancer deaths.[3] The United States Department of Health and Human Services found that smoking is accountable for 90 percent of lung cancers in men and 79 percent in women.[4] Smoking is a major cause of lung, larynx (voice box), oral cavity, pharynx (throat), esophagus, and bladder cancers, and contributes to stomach, cervix, kidney, and pancreas cancers, as well as some leukemias. A smoker's risk of developing these cancers increases with the number of cigarettes smoked each day, the age smoking was commenced, and the amount of the smoker's lifetime that was spent smoking. Think of the reduction in lung cancer deaths attributed to smoking if smokers would heed these warnings and give up the habit. Significant medical and scientific research is available publicizing the health benefits of smoking cessation.[5, 6, 7] Amazingly, almost one person dies every minute from illnesses related to cigarette smoking in the United States. This accounts for about one in five deaths in the United States.[8]

Smoking harms almost every organ of the body, causes or contributes to a range of diseases, and significantly reduces quality of life. Smoking contributes to heart disease, bronchitis, emphysema, stroke, aneurysms, high cholesterol, pneumonia, influenza, the common cold, chronic bowel disease, peptic ulcers, tooth decay, gum disease, osteoporosis, thyroid disease, cataracts, and bronchitis.[9] It is damaging to reproductive health, especially in women. Smoking is linked with reduced fertility, increased risk of miscarriage, premature births, low birth-weight infants, stillbirth, and infant death.[10, 11, 12, 13, 14] Smoking is a detriment to physical fitness and endurance, because it reduces the ability of the blood to carry oxygen.[15, 16] The American Cancer Society estimates that male chronic smokers lose an average of 13.2 years of life expectancy, while female chronic smokers lose 14.5.[17] Taking into account current (as of 2009 statistics) average life expectancy of 78.5 years in the United States,[18] this equals approximately 17 to 18 percent of a smoker's life.

Instead of dying as a direct result of smoking, many people suffer through life with a debilitating chronic illness, which significantly reduces their quality of life. These people may have to carry an oxygen tank everywhere they go to provide sufficient oxygen to the body. They may suffer from coronary heart disease or stroke. A smoker's quality of life is often reduced during the "golden years," if not earlier.

Ironically, people smoke despite the immediate detrimental effects that are felt when smoking for the first time. A person's first use of tobacco generally causes illness. The body attempts to rid itself of nicotine through expulsion, including coughing and vomiting. As the person smokes more cigarettes and nicotine is continually introduced to the body, a tolerance is built up. Once body tolerance sets in, addiction is likely.[19, 20]

THE SUPERFLUITY OF CHEMICALS IN CIGARETTES LOOMING TO HARM YOUR HEALTH

The three chemicals contained in cigarettes that are most worrisome appear to be nicotine, tar, and carbon monoxide. According to the University of Minnesota, nicotine is as addictive as heroin, 1,000 times more potent than alcohol and 5 to 10 times more potent than cocaine and morphine.[21] Tar is a resinous particulate produced when burning tobacco that accumulates in the smoker's lungs and can lead to lung cancer and other ailments. Ironically, we increasingly place carbon monoxide detectors in our homes to avoid exposure to this toxic killer, yet we allow people to inhale it in cigarettes everyday. How many of us would line up to inhale exhaust from a pipe connected to a car's exhaust system before the catalytic converter—where the majority of the carbon monoxide is eliminated? Yet smokers voluntarily introduce the same toxic chemical into their bodies through smoking cigarettes. Carbon monoxide is a silent killer we should strive to avoid in any form.

Many of the chemicals that are used in various industries are found in cigarettes. We wear protective equipment to avoid exposure to these chemicals, but they are easily accessible in cigarettes. It is curious that government agencies fine industries and employers for allowing employees to come in unprotected contact with the same chemicals found in cigarettes yet allow smokers to inhale them every day. One would think that cigarettes would be banned outright, or at least controlled more ardently given the many of harmful chemicals contained in them. I believe an employer would find it hard to convince the Occupational Safety Hazard Association that their employees would be safe coming in contact with the same plethora of chemicals during the workday.

Rather than bore you with scientific data about all four thousand chemicals in cigarettes, I will give a brief overview of a few of the most harmful chemicals they contain.

Tar, a sticky black by-product of burning tobacco, clogs the lungs and may cause lung cancer. Some of the carcinogenic (cancer causing) chemicals contained in tar are

- **Benzopyrene:** This chemical, when exposed to benzopyrene in the short term, has been shown to cause red blood cell damage, leading to anemia, and suppresses the immune system. Long-term exposure has the potential to cause reproductive and developmental damage, and cancer.[22]

- **B-Naphthylamine:** Used in the manufacture of dyes and rubber, this product causes kidney, liver, and brain damage.

- **Cadmium:** This element is extremely poisonous and commonly found in manufacturing facilities where car batteries are made or where ore is smelted or processed. Even trace amounts of this metal can produce harmful effects. Acute inhalation may result in long-lasting impairment of lung function, while chronic exposure can result in kidney, lung, liver, bone, immune system, blood, and nervous system damage.[23]

- **Tobacco-Specific N-Nitrosamine:** In animal studies, nitrosamines are considered one of the most powerful carcinogens. While more research needs to be conducted regarding their full effects on humans, I believe it is safe to say that nitrosamines are unhealthful for humans as well. They have been linked to oral, lung, liver, pancreatic, and esophageal cancer.[24]

Nicotine, a poisonous alkaloid, is the addictive drug contained within cigarettes. Nicotine travels through the bloodstream and to the brain in a matter of seconds. This powerful drug is a stimulant that raises heart rate and blood pressure and increases the stickiness of blood vessels, which in turn increases the risk of heart attack and stroke. Nicotine creates a terrible physical and psychological addiction. Many people attempt to quit smoking each year, but fewer than 5 percent succeed.[25] The physical and emotional addictions of this drug are extremely difficult to overcome. Despite knowing the injurious effects of this habit, smokers have great difficulty quitting. Their addiction becomes more powerful than their desire to live a healthful life and reduce risk of disease. Smokers certainly have not been helped by cigarette manufacturers. According to one report, these "conspiring men" have knowingly and deliberately increased the nicotine levels in cigarettes.[26] Of course, the tobacco industry vehemently denies this allegation, but they also denied that their products were addictive and unhealthy until they were forced to admit it.

Carbon monoxide is not only found in car exhaust but also in cigarette smoke. This deadly poison robs the muscles, brain, and body tissues of oxygen, causing your heart to work harder. This overworking of the heart can cause heart attack and stroke, and over time causes swelling of the airways, letting less air into the lungs. Carbon monoxide is an odorless and colorless gas, making it a silent killer. At lower levels of exposure, carbon monoxide causes headache, dizziness, nausea, fatigue, and disorientation.[27] Carbon monoxide starves your tissues of oxygen by creating carboxyhemoglobin in the blood. At moderate concentrations it may cause angina (heart pain), impaired vision, and reduced brain function. Very high concentrations can be fatal.[28]

How many of us would line up to ingest chemicals used as household cleaning products and fertilizers? Yet this is what smokers do through the inhalation of ammonia contained in cigarettes. Ammonia is an eye, nose, skin, and throat irritant and can cause asthma, acute lung damage, and blindness.[29] Unfortunately, the cigarette companies use ammonia to boost the impact of nicotine in cigarettes. This process of adding ammonia to cigarettes is similar to the process of using chemicals to heighten the effects of cocaine, called "free-basing." Ammonia helps convert nicotine from its acid to base form, allowing it to more fully and quickly circulate through the body. The cigarette companies know that nicotine is the addictive chemical in cigarettes and make it more addictive through this process. Again, this is done without regard to health consequences, simply to increase the salability of the product and profits. The more addicted smokers that can be created, the more profit that is produced.

Arsenic is a naturally occurring compound used in ammunition manufacturing to make bullets harder and rounder. It is used in tanning and taxidermy as a preservative, and as a wood surface preservative and treatment. Much concern has been expressed over the use of arsenic in the treatment of wood used in playground equipment. Industries that use this compound must take great care to avoid exposure and the adverse health affects associated with it. It has been shown to cause diarrhea, nausea, abdominal pain, central and peripheral nervous system disorders, skin and mucous membrane irritation, anemia, peripheral neuropathy, skin lesions, kidney and liver damage, and lung, liver, and bladder cancer.[30]

Benzene is a highly flammable, colorless liquid found in coal and oil burning emissions, gasoline at service stations, and car exhaust. It has a very high melting point and a sweet odor. It has been used as a gasoline additive, pesticide, detergent, dye, lubricant, degreaser, and in explosives. In fact, this toxic chemical was also used to decaffeinate coffee at one point. Benzene may cause drowsiness; dizziness; headaches; eye, skin, and respiratory irritation; unconsciousness, a reduced number of red blood cells; female reproductive harm; and elevate incidences of leukemia (cancer of the tissues that form white blood cells).[31]

Cadmium is a soft transitional metal largely used in batteries and pigments and as a plastic stabilizer. Cadmium exposure may cause a number of harmful health effects in humans, including irritation and damage of the lungs, death, kidney damage, and the formation of kidney stones.[32] In animal studies cadmium has been shown to cause high blood pressure, iron-poor blood, liver disease, and nerve and brain damage.[33]

Chloroform was originally used as an anesthetic during surgery in the mid-1800s. Soon after its use, sudden deaths during anesthesia were reported. Because of these reports and with the advent of safer anesthetics, chloroform fell out of favor. Chloroform is also used in laundry starch, paint-related products, automotive chemicals, pesticides, and specialty cleaning and sanitation products. The predominant use today is for the production of air conditioning refrigerant, but recent environmental legislation will reduce and eliminate this use as refrigerants become more environmentally friendly.[34] Unfortunately, chloroform can be released into the air as a result of its formation in chlorinated drinking water and swimming pools. Its major health effect is central nervous system depression, but it also may cause liver problems (including hepatitis, tumors, and jaundice) and kidney tumors.[35]

Formaldehyde, the same chemical morticians use to embalm deceased individuals, is also found in cigarettes. It is a colorless gas with a pungent odor. The various forms of formaldehyde are used as a preservative and disinfectant and in pressed wood products (its highest concentration level), foam insulation, carpets, clothing, and some appliances. It can cause watery, burning eyes and a burning sensation in the throat. In addition, it can cause nausea, seizures, coma, liver and kidney damage, headache, central nervous system damage, and dermatitis.[36] Animal studies have demonstrated effects on the lungs, spleen, liver, and thyroid and increased incidence of lung, nasal cavity, and liver tumors.[37]

Lead remains one of the greatest environmental health hazards in the United States. It is most dangerous to children because of the likelihood that they will touch a lead object and then put their hands in their mouths. In addition, children seem to absorb lead more readily than adults, and their developing brain and nervous system are more susceptible to its damaging effects.[38] The government banned the use of leaded gasoline to protect us from exposure, but it continues to allow cigarettes that contain lead to be sold. Regrettably, toys manufactured in China have been exposed for the use of lead-based paint. That a manufacturer would allow toys that will without a doubt end up in children's mouths to be coated with a deadly toxin is unconscionable. But, then again, the cigarette industry does the same thing—knowingly supplying a lead-containing product that ultimately ends up in the mouths of adults. Lead is primarily used in the manufacture of lead-acid storage batteries, but it is also used in alloys, ammunition, and foil, as cable coverings, in the lining of laboratory sinks, and in the protective shielding against x-ray and radiation. It may cause brain and nervous system damage, behavior and learning disabilities, hyperactivity, impeded growth, hearing problems, headaches, reproductive problems (both men and women), high blood pressure, nerve disorders, memory and concentration problems, and muscle and joint pain.[39]

Vinyl chloride is primarily used in the production of PVC (polyvinyl chloride) plastic and vinyl products. It was once used as an aerosol spray propellant in products like hairspray and briefly as an inhalational anesthetic, though this practice was discontinued when its toxicity was discovered. Exposure to vinyl chloride can result in central nervous system problems such as dizziness, drowsiness, and headaches, and other health effects like liver damage and cancer.[40]

THE FAR-REACHING EFFECTS OF
SECONDHAND SMOKE (ETS)

Sadly, those who choose to smoke don't just affect themselves but also anyone else who is exposed to the by-product of their smoking, secondhand smoke, or environmental tobacco smoke (ETS). Smokers are so addicted to their habit that they often expose someone they love and care about to ETS. I am dismayed when I see an adult smoking in the front seat of their car, with their children in the backseat. Either they don't care, or don't understand, the negative consequences of this practice. With all the media regarding the negative effects of smoking, the former is more likely. Apparently their addiction to cigarettes is more powerful than the love they have for their family or friends.

ETS comes in two forms, sidestream smoke (smoke from the end of a lit cigarette, cigar, or pipe) and mainstream smoke (smoke exhaled by the smoker). This involuntary smoking, forced upon virtually everyone, exposes unwilling victims to the same superfluity of toxic, noxious, and harmful chemicals smokers are exposed to. Disappointingly, many smokers choose to smoke near playgrounds, schools, parks, and other locations frequented by children. As children play hard and breathe heavily, they become the unfortunate recipients of significant levels of ETS.

ETS is classified as a known human carcinogen by the Environmental Protection Agency (EPA), International Agency for Research on Cancer (IARC), a division of the World Health Organization (WHO), and the United States National Toxicology Program.[41] ETS can linger in the air long after the source has been extinguished and can cause or exacerbate many adverse health effects, including cancer, respiratory infections, and asthma.[42] Exposure to ETS can ultimately lead to disease and death among those who do not smoke. In fact ETS causes 3,400 lung cancer deaths and 46,000 heart disease deaths in nonsmokers in the United States each year.[43] This is an astounding fact and should give us all reason to fight for greater rights for nonsmokers. Eliminating exposure to ETS and avoiding this assault should be a conscious effort for all of us. The best protection would be to ban tobacco products outright. Unfortunately, this is extremely unlikely to happen, so the next best thing would be to limit smoking to the smoker's place of residence. Again, not likely to happen; the rights of the few seem to outweigh the rights of the majority with regard to this issue. Governments are willing to overlook this problem as they receive millions of dollars in cigarette taxes.

ETS is especially harmful to children under the age of eighteen months, among whom it is responsible for up to 300,000 lower respiratory infections, 15,000 hospitalizations, and 430 cases of sudden infant death syndrome each year.[44] Shamefully, 21 million children in the United States live in homes where they are exposed to ETS on a regular basis.[45] Should smokers then be held civilly and criminally responsible for these illnesses and deaths? Is this not a form of child abuse? They are in fact willingly and knowingly exposing their children and the children of others to a harmful and sometimes deadly substance. How would a person be treated if they knowingly exposed their children to other toxic substances that resulted in injury or death? There simply is no safe or risk-free level of exposure to ETS. Each time you unwillingly inhale ETS you are risking adverse health effects. The surgeon general reported that even short-term exposure to ETS can cause significant problems with blood vessels, blood platelets, and heart function, potentially increasing heart attack risk.[46]

Lost productivity in the workplace is another consequence of smoking. Not only do smokers take several breaks per day to smoke, but they also tend to be less healthy and require more sick time off than those who don't smoke. The Campaign for Tobacco Free Kids estimates annual productivity loss related to smoking in the United States to be 97.6 billion dollars per year.[47] Smokers also experience decreased value of homes and vehicles as well as greater costs for health and life insurance.

IS SMOKELESS TOBACCO LESS HARMFUL THAN CIGARETTES?

Some smokers quit smoking and instead use what they feel is a more "healthful" form of tobacco: smokeless tobacco, also known as chew. The truth is smokeless tobacco products are not a safe or harmless substitute for cigarettes, cigars, or pipe smoking and are in fact more harmful to your mouth. Smokeless tobacco is linked with oral and pancreatic cancer, leukoplakia (sores in the mouth that can lead to cancer), receding gums, bone loss around the roots of the teeth, teeth abrasions, teeth staining, and bad breath.[48] Smokeless tobacco still contains over twenty known carcinogens,[49] and many other chemicals, including the addictive drug nicotine and high levels of tobacco-specific nitrosamines.[50] The longer a person uses smokeless tobacco products, the more likely they are to have mouth problems, including leukoplakia. This is also a repulsive habit in appearance. The person has a distended appearance to the lips and must expel the chew at some point, often in a can, or worse, on the ground.

MEDICINAL USE OF TOBACCO

It is wise to leave the tobacco products to the uses that the Lord recommends, as a bruise–healing herb and for sick cattle. But even then it must be used with great caution and prudence. Tobacco appears to have medicinal properties for sick animals and has its place when used appropriately. Dr. Rulon Francis conducted experiments with rats and the healing affects of tobacco juice on deliberately inflicted bruises after Brigham Young University's athletic department returned from the Balkan Games in Yugoslavia with stories that trainers had used tobacco spray on basketball player's bruises. His study concluded that the rat group that was treated with the tobacco had 20 percent more healing cells than those rats treated with distilled water only.[51]

TOBACCO USE DESTROYS THE BODY AND SPIRIT

Staying clear of this powerful and debilitating herb is vitally important to maintain health. The use of tobacco products among Church members led the prophet Joseph Smith to inquire of the Lord regarding this practice. Through this inquiry, we received the Word of Wisdom and the Lord's definitive answer and guidance that tobacco is not for man. Tobacco products should be abstained from and are unquestionably harmful to the body. President George A. Smith said, "In my judgment the use of tobacco, as little a thing as it seems to some men, has been the means of destroying their spiritual life, has been the means of driving from them the companionship of the Spirit of the Father, has alienated them from the society of good men and women, and has brought upon them disregard and reproach of the children that have been born to them."[52] Obviously cigarette smoking has drastic affects on spiritual well-being as well as physical well-being.

4

Wholesome Herbs Ordained *for* Man

And again, verily I say unto you, all wholesome herbs God hath ordained for the constitution, nature, and use of man.

Doctrine and Covenants 89:10

This verse is particularly important to me because I believe it was an answer to prayer and ultimately changed my life. After experiencing persistent lower back pain for months, I decided to get it checked out by a doctor. My doctor and the findings of a subsequent rheumatologist confirmed that I had a chronic joint disease called ankylosing spondylitis (AS). The rheumatologist prescribed the normal regimen of prescription medicines, namely prescription strength nonsteroidal anti-inflammatory drugs (NSAIDs), muscle relaxers, and prescription painkillers. At first, it provided great relief from the pain I suffered in my lower back. I thought that I had seen the end of my problems, but in reality they had only just begun. I began experiencing a common side effect of NSAIDs, severe stomach discomfort. The stomach pains were so excruciating that I wondered which pain was worse, my back or stomach pain. I discussed the problem with my doctor, and he offered an additional prescription, a drug to reduce production of acid in the stomach. This only brought temporary relief of the stomach pain I was feeling, and within a couple weeks the stomach pain had returned. At this point, I felt I needed to make a decision between my back pain and my stomach pain, choosing to deal with the lesser of two pains. In addition, my immune system seemed weaker, another common side effect of the prescribed medications. I was susceptible to any illness I was exposed to, and my overall sense of well-being felt reduced.

As trials and hardships often do, this ordeal made me turn to the Lord for help. I didn't want to live with the back pain, but I knew I couldn't continue with the stomach pain either. As I pondered and prayed for guidance, the Word of Wisdom kept coming to mind. I read the Word of Wisdom more carefully than I have ever before and I was impressed that this part of verse 10 was my answer: "all wholesome herbs God hath ordained for the constitution, nature, and use of man." This led me to seek herbs for the two health conditions I was now dealing with. I fortunately happened upon research relating to deglycyrrhizinated licorice root (DGL). This proven remedy for all kinds of stomach and intestinal ulcers did the trick. My stomach pain was relieved quickly, and best of all it was a permanent solution. The DGL repaired the damage the NSAIDs had done to my stomach lining.

With my stomach pain relieved, I completed further research to find natural means to manage my AS. I moved forward with a conviction and belief in herbs and their healing power. I had faith and was sure that I would find an herb, or herbs, to help me with my back condition. After much research, I indeed found a combination of herbs and nutrients that have helped tremendously. I no longer take nor need the NSAIDs that created further health problems. I have been able to manage my illness better with herbs than with prescription medications and avoid the severe side effects. Furthermore, my overall health and well-being have improved. I have increased immunity to illness and feel more vitality.

HERBS AS MEDICINE

Some revealing words are contained within this scripture. One dictionary states the medical meaning of *constitution* is "the physical makeup of the body; including its functions, metabolic processes, reactions to stimuli, and resistance to the attack of pathogenic organisms."[1]

Another dictionary defines constitution as "the physical makeup of the individual especially with respect to health, strength, and appearance of the body; the structure, composition, physical makeup, or nature of something." We are told that man was formed from the dust of the earth, and man must have the "dust," or elements, of the earth replenished in the body repeatedly to avoid ill health. Our Father in Heaven is telling us this when He used the word *constitution*. We need to understand that our bodies require elements from the earth to survive, and the best way to get these elements is through plants. The word *herb* refers to plants that are beneficial to and healthful for man. Plants store nutrients they draw from the soil and the air, including vitamins and minerals. When we consume plants, we gain these nutrients and use them to build up our bodies. Plants and herbs can regulate the functions and metabolic processes of the body, and that is their intention. God put them on the earth for our benefit and this purpose.

The word *wholesome* is also important. According to TheFreeDictionary.com, *wholesome* means healthy, completeness, the state of being whole. Every plant God has created contains its peak nutrients, including vitamins and minerals, in whole form. This is the form God intends us to eat them in because in this state we receive the most benefit from available nutrients. We must also distinguish between wholesome and harmful herbs. Marijuana is an herb, but it is not wholesome and therefore should be avoided. Not everything that is natural is wholesome, nor safe. A word of caution regarding the use of herbs. Herbal usage requires skill and study, so it is best to consult a qualified practitioner before self-treatment. Some herbs and even vitamins and minerals can interact with or interfere with medications, leading to unintended consequences.

Ordained is another keyword. It means to establish or order by decree or law.[2] All things upon this earth were created by God and work according to His laws and within His order. Being thus, plants will work according to God's purpose inside the human body. When eaten in their unadulterated form, plant foods will promote a healing effect from within and stimulate the proper function of vital organs and biological processes. All of this is completed in a safe and gentle manner. God in his infinite wisdom has placed on earth all the nutrient-rich plants we need to stay healthy. I am convinced God has placed herbs for the benefit of most conditions and diseases known to man on earth.

THE MEDICINAL USE OF HERBS
THROUGHOUT HISTORY

Herbs have been used throughout recorded history, and in all likelihood started with Adam and Eve. A conversation between Adam and Eve and God is recorded in the Bible as "And God said, Behold, I have given you every herb bearing seed, which is upon the face of all the earth, and every tree, in the which is the fruit of a tree yielding seed; to you shall be for meat" (Genesis 1:29). Similar accounts are recorded in Moses 2:29 and Abraham 4:29. Adam and Eve were given instruction to utilize the herbs and fruits of the trees available to them for their "meat." This includes the use as both food and medicine. In Ezekiel 47:12 we read, "and the fruit thereof shall be for meat and the leaves thereof for medicine." This is another acknowledgment of the importance of using herbs as our medicine. Many plant leaves are used in medicinal teas, ground up and encapsulated, or turned into a tincture.

Ancient civilizations relied upon herbs as medicine, food, perfume, disinfectants, and sometimes as currency. Ancient records, including the Bible, tell us that the Egyptians, Chinese, Greeks, Romans, and other societies all knew of and used the medicinal power of herbs. Hippocrates, an early Greek physician before the time of Christ, developed a system of medicine utilizing herbs.[3] The Nephites were another ancient civilization well versed in the use of herbs as medicine. In Alma 46:40, we read "And there were some who died with fevers, which at some seasons of the year were very frequent in the land—but not so much so with fevers, because of the excellent qualities of the many plants and roots which God had prepared to remove the cause of disease, to which men were subject by the nature of the climate." Herbs were used to treat these fevers and "remove the cause of disease" among the Nephites. They knew the power of herbs and used them with great skill to benefit their people.

HERBAL MEDICINE AMONG THE
EARLY AND MODERN-DAY SAINTS

Herbal medicine was also commonly used among the early Saints. The Newel K. Whitney store was known to have stocked foodstuffs, textiles, household and hardware goods, books, and herbal medicines. Brigham Young wrote a letter to the Mormon Battalion that contained the following advice:

A letter from Brigham Young:

Camp of Israel, Omaha Nation

Cutler's Park

August 19th, 1846

To Captain Jefferson Hunt and the Captains, Officers, and Soldiers of the Mormon Battalion.

We have the opportunity of sending to Fort Leavenworth this morning by Dr. Reed a package of twenty-five letters, which we improve, with his word of counsel to you all: If you are sick, live by faith, and let the surgeon's medicine alone. If you want to live, [use] only such herbs and mild food as are at your disposal. If you give heed to this counsel, you will prosper; but if not, we cannot be responsible for the consequences. A hint to the wise is sufficient.

In behalf of the council,

Brigham Young, President[4]

Another discourse from Brigham Young affirms his belief in people being responsible for their own health and the health of their families, as well as the significance of herbs in this care. He said, "It is God's mind and will that they [every father and mother] should know just what to do for them [their children] when they are sick. Instead of calling for a doctor you should administer to them by the laying on of hands and anointing them with oil, and give them mild food, and herbs, and medicine that you understand."[5] Parents have the primary responsibility and are the primary caregivers for their children. This includes caring for them when sick as much as they have means and knowledge to do so.

Subsequent presidents of the Church have also declared their belief in the healing power of herbs. In 1982, President Spencer W. Kimball stated, "We should do all we can for ourselves first: dieting, resting, taking simple herbs known to be effective, and applying common sense, especially to minor trouble."[6] Currently, pediatricians are overloaded with parents who bring their children to the doctor for simple ailments such as colds. Often the doctor feels obligated to provide an antibiotic so the parents don't feel like the trip and their money was wasted, despite the fact that colds are caused by a virus, which antibiotics don't work against. Unfortunately, this contributes to disease-resistant bacteria—so called superbugs—and perpetuates the myth that we have to take our children to the doctor for every simple ailment.

THE INNATE HEALING POWER OF THE BODY

In fact, most acute ailments can be healed by the body alone if it is allowed the opportunity. This includes consuming only mild foods and drinking plenty of clean water. Herbs are used to stimulate biological processes within a person, thus allowing the body to heal itself. They enhance the body's innate and natural ability to heal. An example of this innate ability is a cut on your arm. If it has no foreign object in it and the cut is kept clean and free of bacteria, it will heal itself. On the other hand, if an natural ointment of aloe vera or calendula is applied, the wound-healing process will be enhanced. Nothing can increase the speed of the healing process within the body greater than its capabilities. The body will only heal as fast as it is designed. However, herbs and other natural methods provide the optimal environment and nourishment for the speediest healing to take place.

THE SAFETY AND EFFICACY OF PLANT-BASED REMEDIES

Herbs are not like the synthetic chemicals that are most modern medicines. Though many modern medicines originate from plants and herbs, they are in an adulterated form. Man takes the active constituent (the one that is active biochemically and appears to have the most substantial affect) of the plant and removes it from the hundreds of other constituents contained within the plant to use it as medicine. This is an unnatural state. Man, in his arrogance, removes the protective constituents that God intended in the whole form of the plant, thus increasing or causing negative side effects associated with the one "active" constituent. Herbs promote the natural functions of the body with the hundreds of biochemical constituents they contain. God is the creator of all herbs, and no man can match His knowledge of chemistry and biology, thus it is foolish to believe that we can create synthetic chemicals that will function better than the herbs God created.

Herbs are tremendously safe when used by a skilled herbalist, or one knowledgeable in the usage of herbs. It is incongruous that the US Food and Drug Administration is so prone to censure the effectiveness and safety of herbs, while promoting prescription drugs as safe and effective. A comparison of the safety of herbs versus prescription drugs establishes a clear picture. Prescription drugs are estimated to cause 106,000 deaths and an astonishing 2,216,000 serious adverse drug reactions annually in the United States.[7] Compare these astounding statistics to that of herbs and dietary supplements. In a twenty-three-year period, 1.6 million exposures to harmful substances were reported to poison control. An exposure is defined as a call to the poison control center reporting actual or potential exposure to a substance.[8] It is possible the exposure didn't even occur. In addition, the exposure does not indicate the person experienced any negative effects as a result of the exposure. Of these 1.6 million exposures, it was reported that 251,799 of these cases required hospitalization.[9] In twenty-two years, only 230 deaths have been reported as a result of dietary supplements, or about 10 per year.[10] I find it interesting that the author of a dietary supplement essay that includes these figures decries this report when by his own numbers prescription drugs are almost nine times more likely to cause an adverse reaction, and over ten thousand times more likely to be fatal.[11]

THE FAILURES OF MODERN MEDICINE

We have to ask ourselves why the FDA does little to protect the public from poisonous and deadly drugs while devoting significant attention to "protecting" the public from safe herbs. It seems lately that every month there is another prescription drug, previously approved for use by the FDA, being pulled from the shelves because of adverse reactions and deaths associated with its proper use. Maybe the FDA should spend more time investigating and evaluating the real threat to the American public: prescription drugs.

It is ironic that despite the United States having one of the most sophisticated and technologically advanced systems of medicine in the world, it ranks last among industrialized nations in preventable deaths.[12] This is mostly because the US health care system does not practice primary preventative medicine, it practices sick care. The US medical system chooses to focus on early detection methods rather than primary preventative measures like diet, environmental, and lifestyle factors. Medical students receive little, if any, courses aimed at better understanding nutrition and lifestyle factors that contribute to disease. Instead they are indoctrinated in the "pill or surgery for every ill" myth. The American public in many ways demands this. We do not wish to change our lifestyles and diets in order to maintain or improve our health. Instead we ask for the newest surgery or pill to save us from our poor choices. We want, and our scientists and doctors seek, the "miracle" cure for cancer, arthritis, diabetes, and so on, rather than learning to prevent these diseases. Maybe this is because it is easier, or maybe it is due to the lack of education and information provided to the American public in this regard. If our physicians are not receiving this knowledge from the medical schools, how are they to teach others about it? Knowledge truly is power, and the more education we can empower the general public with, the healthier we will become.

Another study places the United States as forty-fifth among average life expectancy at birth.[13] Many of the countries above the US in the study maintain better diets and integrate more natural therapies, including herbs, into their health care systems, which focus more on preventative care. These countries take a more proactive approach to health care, whereas the US system is reactive. These countries also tend to have more active lifestyles when compared to the inhabitants of the United States.

The US health care system is also hesitant or unwilling to integrate natural healing methods. Other countries utilize herbs, nutrition, vitamins and minerals, and lifestyle factors as integrative and all-encompassing approach to health care. Meanwhile, US physicians continue to rely upon drugs and surgery almost exclusively. These options are far more invasive than those used by other countries. An example of this is St. John's wort, an herb often used in other countries to treat mild to moderate depression with few side effects.[14, 15] In fact, several recent studies suggest side effects occur in only 1–3 percent of patients taking this beneficial herb.[16] On the other hand, the monoamineoxidase inhibitor (MAOI) drugs that are predominantly used in the US for the treatment of depression carry with them a superfluity of adverse side effects, including a higher rate of suicide among teenagers.[17] Fifty percent of patients that take MAOIs experience some kind of adverse reaction to them. This means these patients are sixteen to fifty times more likely to experience a negative effect while taking MAOIs versus St. John's wort.

This unfortunate reality is largely due to the power and influence of the multibillion-dollar prescription drug manufacturers. They invest billions of dollars in advertising and medical schools and shower doctors with gifts and incentives to push their products. In my opinion, these manufacturers are another group of "evil and conspiring men." They don't want to investigate the safety and effectiveness of herbs, nor promote them as treatments because they can't patent an herb that God manufactured. There simply aren't the same billions of dollars to be made in dietary supplements as there are in expensive drugs.

Now this does not meant that every prescription drug is bad and herbs have a corner on the healing market, nor does it mean that modern medicine should be abolished. Herbs and natural treatments should be used complementary with modern medicine. There is not one system of health that has the complete answer to every human ailment and disease. What we do know is that there are safer alternatives to many prescription drugs and surgeries currently being utilized by US physicians. There are also times when a prescription drug is appropriate, like during acute, life-threatening situations. In general, because herbs work with the body and stimulate the power within the body to heal, they act more slowly than prescription drugs. It would therefore be unwise to wait for this action to take place during an acute, life-threatening situation. Technology to diagnose disease is also beneficial. A proper diagnosis is often key in determining the best course of action to take in regards to disease treatment. Many advances have also been made that go beyond the scope of herbal healing. All beneficial treatments should be combined and utilized in health care, with a preference for the most noninvasive, safe, and effective treatments. US physicians and especially medical schools would be wise to more open-mindedly investigate complementary treatments that are less invasive and harmful to the American public.

THE INEFFICIENCIES OF THE CURRENT
UNITED STATES HEALTH CARE SYSTEM

Health care costs are growing at a deplorable rate in the United States. Insurance costs have consistently risen at a much higher rate than inflation or wages. In 2005, health care expenditures rose 6.9 percent, or twice that of inflation.[18] Many Americans are without health insurance not because they choose not to carry it, but because they can't afford it. Nearly 47 million Americans are uninsured.[19] Health care spending is 4.3 times the amount spent on our national defense[20] and equals about $6,700 per person, amounting to two *trillion* dollars in 2005.[21] These costs and expenditures could be reduced with the integration of herbs and dietary supplements into the US health care system. Going back to our St. John's wort/MAOI example, St. John's wort is a fraction of the cost of MAOI drugs. This is but one example, and there are many other supplements proven effective in managing disease that could be implemented at significant cost savings. Regretfully, this is unlikely to happen as the deep pockets of the pharmaceutical companies would not be padded with herbs as they have been with prescription drugs. There simply is not the same financial incentive in herbs as there is in prescription drugs. Again, "conspiring men" care more about profit than they do the health of millions of Americans.

Our health care system is riddled with inefficiencies, unnecessary and excessive tests, excessive administrative fees, inflated prices, waste, and fraud. One must ask if the United States has the best health care system, or simply the most expensive. The statistics seem to support the latter. If more effective and safe natural remedies were utilized in the US, how much money could our health care system save? How many lives could be improved upon or saved? We may never know the answer to these questions.

5

Fruits *and* Vegetables

Every herb in the season thereof, and every fruit in the season thereof; all these to be used with prudence and thanksgiving.

All grain is good for the food of man; as also the fruit of the vine; that which yieldeth fruit, whether in the ground or above the ground.

Doctrine & Covenants 89:11, 16

Fruits and vegetables should make up the bulk of the diet, particularly vegetables. We would be wise to notice the important health benefits of fruits and vegetables. Most fruits and vegetables are low in fat and calories, and none contain cholesterol. They are high in potassium and fiber, both important nutrients to maintain a healthy body. Diets high in potassium may help control blood pressure, and dietary fiber helps reduce cholesterol, reducing the risk of heart disease.[1,2] Fiber also acts as a sponge, soaking up cholesterol and sending it for elimination through the bowel.

THE HUMAN HEALTH BENEFITS OF PLANT, VEGETABLE, AND FRUIT PHYTONUTRIENTS

In order to take full advantage of the nutrients and phytonutrients—biologically active compounds found in plants that provide health-protecting and health-promoting benefits to humans—fruits and vegetables contain, eat a variety of colors. Each vegetable or fruit has its own makeup of beneficial vitamins, minerals, and other nutrients. These vitamins and minerals regulate body functions and facilitate chemical reactions within the body. It is best to add as much diversity as possible when eating fruits and vegetables in order to gain the maximum benefit from their disease-preventing phytonutrients. The skins of fruits and vegetables are particularly important because they hold many of these vital nutrients.

Vegetables provide the broadest range of phytochemicals, vitamins, and minerals of any food group. Dark-green vegetables like spinach, broccoli, and romaine lettuce contain nutrients that are beneficial to the bones, lungs, immune system, and brain.[3] Orange vegetables like carrots, pumpkin, and sweet potatoes promote eye health, help maintain blood sugar control, and contain cancer-fighting carotenoids.[4] Starchy vegetables like potatoes and corn contain a unique blend of antioxidants and significant quantities of many vitamins and minerals.[5] The Lord in His infinite wisdom has made a multiplicity and abundance of vegetables each with its own distinctive health benefits.

When fruits and vegetables are eaten in their unrefined, unprocessed, fresh, and natural state, a large portion of the carbohydrates are "complex." Complex carbohydrates provide a significant amount of fiber, phytonutrients, vitamins, minerals, enzymes, and usable energy for the body. God intended us to receive all of the nutrients from these wholesome foods. Complex carbohydrates are digested more slowly, curtailing large swings in blood sugar. Keep in mind that the more you cook fruits or vegetables, the more nutrients and phytochemicals you destroy—particularly the enzymes intended to help you digest and absorb their nutrients. Soaking vegetables in water removes some of the nutrients into the water and should be avoided unless your intent is to drink the water as well. Overcooking also changes the flavor of vegetables.

THE HEALTH BENEFITS OF EATING AMPLE FRUITS AND VEGETABLES

Studies have found that those who eat the most fruits and vegetables as part of their regular diet have lower risk of coronary heart disease,[6, 7] and stroke.[8] In addition, the regular consumption of fruits and vege-tables as part of a healthy diet may reduce the risk of type 2 diabetes and protect against certain cancers.[9, 10] Because most vegetables are low in fat and calories and none have cholesterol, eating them in place of high-calorie, high-fat, high-cholesterol foods results in more protection against obesity and other chronic illnesses. Most vegetables and fruits promote an alkaline blood environment. Alkaline blood is more disease and infection resistant. Disease-causing agents like bacteria and viruses prefer and require an acidic environment to thrive in.

Most people should strive to include five to thirteen servings of fruits and vegetables in their diet daily. This may seem a daunting task at first, but it is accomplishable with proper planning and an understanding of what equates a serving. A general guideline to follow is that one half cup is a serving. The exceptions to this rule are lettuce and other leafy greens, which are one full cup per serving, and dried fruit, which are a quarter cup per serving.[11, 12] Fruits and vegetables should be included at every meal and in a wide assortment. Including a broad array stimulates the senses with a diversity of colors, smells, and tastes. No one fruit or vegetable contains all the nutrients a person needs, thus it is prudent to include many in your diet.

The high fiber content found in fruits and vegetables is beneficial to the gastrointestinal system and colon and promotes regular function of the bowel. Because fiber is resistant to digestion, it soaks up water like a sponge as it passes through the digestive system and speeds elimination. This reduces pressure on the intestinal tract and may help prevent con-stipation, diverticuli (development of small, irritable pouches inside the colon), and diverticulitis (the painful inflammation of these pouches). High-fiber foods provide a feeling of fullness with fewer calories. This may help reduce the overall caloric intake in your diet. The natural water and sugar content in fruits and vegetables (especially fruits) speeds metabolism and waste elimination, helping to cleanse the body of toxins and waste.

Eye health is improved with the vitamins and phytonutrients found in vegetables. Vegetables high in vitamin A support night vision, and the carotenoids lutein and zeaxanthin have been shown to accumulate in the eye, providing protection to their sensitive tissues.[13] These carot-enoids are found in abundance in dark-green leafy vegetables and some fruits. When your mother told you to eat your carrots because it would promote healthy vision, she was right. Because of their high vitamin A and carotenoid content, a diet rich in fruits and vegetables may even protect against cataracts and macular degeneration.[14]

Fruits and vegetables that are rich in potassium may help maintain healthy blood pressure.[15] In fact, increasing potassium may be more effective in lowering blood pressure than decreasing sodium intake. Recent studies have shown that decreasing salt intake alone is less effective. Additionally, these fruits and vegetables may reduce the risk of developing kidney stones and decrease bone loss.[16] As an electrolyte, potassium regulates water balance within the body as well as the acid-alkali balance in the blood and tissues. This mineral is important to cellular function and helps generate muscle contractions and regulates the heartbeat. As with most vitamins and minerals, the best way to get this mineral is from your diet, thus requiring a substantial intake of the proper fruits and vegetables.

Another important consideration is the body's acid-alkali balance. The cells of the human body are swimming in a vast amount of liquid that is either acid or alkali. The blood should remain slightly alkaline or neutral to promote optimal health. Internal body functions operate best in a neutral to slightly alkaline environment, while disease thrives in an acidic environment. An alkaline environment is optimal for cellular and metabolic processes. If the fluids of the body shift too far to the acid side, life and health-sustaining biological and cellular processes fail to function properly. Too much acid in bodily fluids also reduces the ability to absorb vitamins and minerals, promotes toxic overload, and decreases immune system function. If this over-acidity begins to take place, the body will protect itself by buffering the acid with alkaline minerals (calcium, magnesium, potassium, and sodium) from the body's mineral reserves. When these reserves are depleted, the body borrows from whatever source it can find, including the bones and vital organs. If this process of borrowing continues for too long, the bones, muscles, and organs are weakened, and poor health can result.[17]

Most experts agree that optimally your diet should be between 65 and 80 percent alkaline. In fact, some reports suggest that cancer cells thrive in an acidic environment and deteriorate in an alkaline environment. Your proper dietary intake will vary depending on many factors. Supplying the body the proper balance of alkaline- and acid-producing foods is important to cellular and total health. The following table provides a short, but far from all encompassing, list of common alkaline-producing and acidic-producing foods.

LOCAL, SEASONAL PRODUCE IS BEST

The Lord gives us important direction when He says "in the season thereof." When we eat fruits and vegetables in season, we eat them at their peak nutrient level. We get their full complement of vitamins, minerals, phytonutrients, enzymes, and fiber—all that God intended us to receive from their consumption. It is best to eat locally grown produce whenever possible, because most produce that is not locally grown is picked before it is fully ripened (thus not fully developed nutritionally) and then shipped to us often from hundreds of miles away. Some of this produce is irradiated (exposed to radiation to disinfect, sanitize, and preserve) during the journey to the grocery store to prevent spoilage and eliminate harmful microorganisms, further depleting nutrients.

The most beneficial way to eat fruits is raw and vegetables raw or steamed. Eating them in this form leaves the majority of the beneficial nutrients intact. Steamed may be the optimal way to eat vegetables because it minimally reduces nutrient content while softening vegetables to make them more digestible. Cooking vegetables reduces their nutrient content, but too many raw vegetables in the diet can cause indigestion and gas.

Despite all the arguments from non-organic farmers to the contrary, the healthiest produce is organic. Organic produce is not laced with chemical pesticides, waxed, or irradiated. Even if non-organic produce is washed, pesticides leach into the skins of the produce, and you consume small quantities of these poisons each time you eat it. If you compare an organic apple to a non-organic apple, the non-organic apple will be more aesthetically appealing. This is due to the wax sprayed on the fruit to make it more attractive. Some fruits are even dyed to make them appear more lush and vibrant. This has nothing to do with taste, only appearance. When you consume the two fruits, the organic apple is crisper and more flavorful. Fruits and vegetables contain a significant quantity of phytonutrients and flavonoids, which have various beneficial biochemical and antioxidant effects. Phytonutrients provide the color, scent, and flavor in vegetables and work within the human body to promote health.

They may even strengthen the immune system. Some believe that citrus fruits have dozens of anti-cancer compounds alone, and studies support this notion.[18, 19, 20, 21] The powerful phytonutrients in fruits and vegetables are beneficial in preventing disease and in normalizing body function and chemistry.

The fruits and vegetables that come in certain seasons contain necessary phytonutrients for that particular season. God intends us to eat these plant foods in the season thereof for us to receive maximum nutritional benefit. This doesn't mean that we can't consume fruits and vegetables out of their normal season, but it does indicate the superiority of nutrients obtained from fruits and vegetables during their normal season. In spring, the earth is replenished after the cold of winter, plants grow and flourish, and earth's full beauty radiates. During this season, we receive greens, vegetables, berries, and fruits to build our bodies back up after being somewhat dormant during the winter months. In the summer, we get melons, fruits, and vegetables that provide the necessary nutrients for our bodies to withstand the heat. Many of these fruits contain significant amounts of water to quench our thirst during the heat of summer. The fall provides plant foods that enable our bodies to prepare for the cold winter ahead. Just before winter arrives, we are able to harvest a variety of foods that will store in a natural and nourishing state and are valuable for our winter diet. Winter is generally a period of less activity, requiring us to monitor more closely the foods we consume to avoid putting on excess weight. The exceptions would be those who live in freezing climates and require extra nutrients to maintain proper body heat and insulation from the cold.

FURTHER HEALTH BENEFITS OF PLANT-BASED NUTRIENTS

Chlorophyll is to the plant as blood is to humans; the plant would die without it. It is used by the plant to absorb sunlight and uses this energy to synthesize carbohydrates. When humans consume chlorophyll, it has a soothing effect on the mucous linings and helps in the detoxification process (particularly the liver). Applied topically, chlorophyll is beneficial for skin ulcers.[22] The lifeblood of plants, chlorophyll appears to have important healing and therapeutic effects on humans.

For a brief description of the primary nutrients (including vitamins, minerals, and phytonutrients) found in common fruits and vegetables, see appendix A. The nutrients are listed in alphabetical order, not by amounts of nutrients. While it is not a complete list of the nutrients these plant foods contain, it does give a good overview. This chart is meant as a guide to help you determine what fruits and vegetables to include in your diet to ensure a well-rounded range of nutrients. Further information can be obtained from the US Department of Agriculture's Food and Nutrition Information Center website.

Make sure to at least peruse the nutrients you are gaining and missing out on based upon the common foods you consume. With a basic idea of what nutrients are available from fruits and vegetables, it is important that you understand what their function within the body is. Appendix B is a summary of the function of the nutrients listed in appendix A. Additionally, the Dietary Reference Intake (DRI) established by the Food and Nutrition Board of the Institute of Medicine is listed. This value is established for a healthy adult, and is considered the amount sufficient to avoid deficiency disease. Please note it doesn't consider the individual nature of human beings nor what is necessary to obtain or maintain optimal health. Your actual needs can and will likely vary greatly from the DRIs.

Common Alkaline and Acidic Foods

Alkaline	Acidic
almonds, apples, apricots, avocados, bananas, beans, broccoli, Brazil nuts, cabbage, carrots, cauliflower, celery, cherries, cucumbers, grapes, green beans, lettuce, mushrooms, onions, peaches, pears, potatoes, raisins, raspberries, soy beans, strawberries, tomatoes, watermelon	bacon, beef, beer, blueberries, bread, butter, cashews, cheese, chicken, chocolate, coffee, cola, eggs, ice cream, lamb, lobster, milk, mustard, oysters, pasta, peanuts, peanut butter, peas, pecans, pork, salmon, sausage, shrimp, soft drinks, sugar, turkey, walnuts

If you reviewed both appendices, you can clearly see the consumption of fruits and vegetables provides a multiplicity of health benefits. There would be less disease and better overall health for mankind if more fruits and vegetables were eaten in place of fatty high-calorie foods. The health of many would be improved if we would snack on fruits and vegetables as a substitute for candy and junk food. It is also obvious that fruits and vegetables exert a powerful effect in the control, management, and reversal of diseases and adverse health conditions.

6

Consume Animal Products Sparingly

Yea, flesh also of beasts and of the fowls of the air, I the Lord, have ordained for the use of man with thanksgiving; nevertheless they are to be used sparingly. And it is pleasing unto me that they should not be used, only in time of winter, or of cold, or famine.

Doctrine and Covenants 89:12–13

It is obvious that the Lord made animals available for our consumption. However, most people read the first portion of this verse indicating it is acceptable to consume animals without regarding the counsel to use them sparingly and in times of cold, winter, or famine. The fact is that the more animal products you consume, the greater your risk for disease. Conversely, the more plant foods you consume the lesser your risk of disease. The average American consumes about eight ounces of meat per day, or over 180 pounds of meat per year.[1] This is significantly more than the two to three ounces per day recommended as part of a healthy diet. Americans that consume high quantities of meat are simply eating themselves to death. Most of us grew up on this diet and may not know how to cook a "meatless" meal. Many studies indicate overconsumption of meat is associated with an increased risk for cancer, diabetes, asthma, arthritis, and heart disease. In fact, an epidemiological study demonstrated that pre-menopausal women who ate more than 3.7 ounces of meat per day increased their risk of breast cancer 12 percent, while consumption below this threshold was associated with a 32 percent decrease in breast cancer risk.[2] Post-menopausal women fared even worse. Even when they consumed low levels of meat, the study indicated a 52 percent increase in breast cancer risk, and high levels of meat consumption increased risk 63 percent.[3] Another study indicated that red meats and processed meats increased colorectal cancer rates up to 35 and 49 percent, accordingly.[4] Red meat has also been associated with significantly elevated risk of esophageal, liver, and lung cancers.[5] That twelve-ounce steak we love to eat at restaurants may be contributing to debilitating diseases that will sneak up on us in the near future.

CHOOSING HEALTHY MEAT OPTIONS

A growing body of evidence suggests that red meat, processed meats, and pork are the worst meats for your health.[6, 7, 8] Healthier meat choices are fish, seafood, turkey, and chicken. Of course, all of these choices can be made worse by the manner in which they are cooked. Frying and smoking meats increases the adverse health effects associated with them. If you choose to include red meats in your diet, purchase lean cuts and try to limit consumption to three ounces of meat per day or less. The human gastrointestinal system's pocketed design is not well suited to eat meat as a significant portion of the human diet. This design coupled with too much meat consumption allows meat to putrefy and decompose in the intestines, promoting an ideal environment for bacteria and pathogens to develop.

Fat is often characterized as something we should avoid entirely in the diet. It has the reputation as the primary contributor to obesity. However, good fats perform many beneficial functions within the body. Fat is a useful source of energy, a more efficient source than protein. Fat plays a role in the absorption of and utilization of the fat-soluble vitamins A, D, E, and K. Fat is a fundamental part of the membrane that surrounds each cell in the body. It also makes up the covering that protects nerve cells and is a structural component of cell membranes in the brain. Fatty acids promote healthy skin and regulate body temperature by nourishing the insulating layer of fat just below the skin. Vital organs, such as the kidneys and heart are surrounded and protected by fat. Additionally, fat adds flavor and taste to food.

HEALTHY FATS

Moderate consumption of fat is healthy and necessary, particularly the right kinds of fat. However, too much fat is a contributing factor in degenerative diseases such as heart disease and diabetes. Moreover, the right type of fat is necessary for the health of the body. The essential fatty acids, omega-3 and omega-6, are necessary for human health. They are considered essential because the body can't manufacture them. This means these important fatty acids must be obtained from food. Most Americans consume way too many omega-6 fatty acids compared to omega-3. A proper balance between these two acids is important to promote optimal health. A healthy diet includes a reduction in saturated fat, trans fat, and omega-6 fatty acids, combined with an increase in omega-3 fatty acids. It simply isn't enough to reduce unhealthy fats from the diet; they must be substituted with healthy fats.

Omega-3 fatty acids are divided into three major categories: alpha-linolenic acid (ALA), eicosapentaenoic acid (EPA), and docosahexaenoic acid (DHA). ALA is converted to EPA then DHA inside the body. These oils are predominantly found in coldwater fish, some nut oils, and certain plants. The benefit of plant-based omega-3 fatty acids is that they generally also contain vitamin E to help prevent rancidity. Omega-3 fatty acids play a vital role in normal growth and development, as well as brain function. Omega-3 fatty acids have been shown to reduce inflammation and reduce the risk of many chronic diseases such as cancer, arthritis, and heart disease. They are highly concentrated within the brain and appear to be important for brain and behavioral function. Deficiency in this fatty acid is a contributing factor in many illnesses.[9, 10]

Omega-6 fatty acids are found in meats and most vegetable oils. They work with omega-3 fatty acids to promote proper brain function and normal growth and development. However, excess consumption of omega-6 fatty acids promotes inflammation and increases risks of many chronic diseases. They should be consumed sparingly.

Another category of fatty acids is omega-9, which isn't really considered an essential fatty acid because the body can produce small amounts of it as long as sufficient quantities of omega-3 and omega-6 fatty acids are present. Olive oil is the best source of omega-9, but it can also be obtained from avocados, almonds, sesame oil, cashews, and more.

FATS TO LIMIT OR AVOID

The kinds of fats that should be particularly avoided or limited are saturated fats and trans fats, or partially hydrogenated fats. Saturated fat is predominantly gained from animal sources and is considered the main dietary cause of high blood cholesterol. Eating too much saturated fat increases the risk of heart disease by promoting the buildup of cholesterol within the arteries. Foods high in saturated fat also contain excessive calories, increasing the chance of obesity. Saturated fat raises bad cholesterol (LDL) and decreases good cholesterol (HDL), thus increasing risk of stroke and atherosclerosis.

Trans fat, or partially hydrogenated fat, is a mostly man-made fat. It is naturally found in small amounts in beef, pork, lamb, and butter fat. It is manufactured by adding hydrogen to vegetable oil through a process called hydrogenation. One might ask why anyone would want to manufacture fat. The reason behind the manufacture of trans fat is a longer shelf life and better flavor stability than other fats. In addition, it is inexpensive to produce, gives food a more desirable taste (addicting people to poor nutritional choices), and adds texture to foods. Just like saturated fats, trans fats raise blood cholesterol, perhaps at a greater rate than saturated fats. Trans fats raise LDL cholesterol and lower HDL cholesterol, increasing the risk of heart disease and stroke. Trans fats are commonly found in potato chips, fried foods, margarine, cookies, pies, and cakes. Recently the government has required food labels to indicate the amount of trans fat a food product contains.

The American Heart Association recommends limiting the amount of saturated fat in the diet to 7 percent and trans fats to 1 percent of total daily calories. For a 2,000-calorie diet, this equates to 140 calories from saturated fat and 20 calories from trans fat, or 16 and 2 grams daily. To put this in perspective, a McDonald's Quarter Pounder with Cheese contains 12 grams saturated fat and 1.5 grams trans fat, and if you include a small fry, you add 1.5 additional grams of saturated fat.[11] If you choose a Burger King Whopper with cheese and small fry instead, you consume 19 grams saturated fat and 4.5 grams trans fat.[12] Incredibly, both of these hamburgers contain more saturated fat than an eight-ounce steak at Sizzler, which checks in at 11 grams saturated fat.[13] Fast food is virtually devoid of nutrients but packed with bad fats, refined sugar, and excessive calories. If you eat either of these meals mentioned above, you would have a difficult time eating two other meals that would not put your intake of bad fats significantly above what is considered healthy. More restaurants are incorporating healthier options to their menus and providing nutritional information, making it easier for consumers to make educated choices. If you do eat out, try to choose healthier alternatives and don't be afraid to ask for nutritional information or make special requests—leave sauces off, exchange fries for a vegetable, and so forth—to make your meal more healthy.

PROTEIN AND YOUR HEALTH

Protein is necessary for many body functions, as has been previously mentioned. Animal products, including dairy, provide a significant amount of protein in the diet. Overconsumption of meat produces excess free radicals that damage the cells of the body. Again, people who eat the most animal-based foods tend to have the most chronic disease. A rodent-based study regarding cancer and protein intake yielded some interesting results. The rodents were dosed with the carcinogen aflatoxin and then fed either a 5 percent or 20 percent protein diet. The rats fed the 20 percent protein diet had significantly higher levels of cancer, while most of those fed the 5 percent protein diet were cancer-free.[14] This suggests that diet, particularly animal protein consumption, plays an important part in cancer initiation. The other interesting finding of this study demonstrated that rodents fed plant proteins, even at high levels, did not experience the same level of cancer as those fed animal protein. In fact, plant-based foods decreased tumor development. It appears that protein from animal sources provides the optimal environment to trigger cancer initiation and growth, while plant proteins do the opposite.

The protein used in this study was the milk protein casein. It is remarkable that human beings are the only mammals that continue to drink milk into adulthood. Milk promotes congestion in the body, depresses the immune system, and some believe it increases the risk of diabetes, heart disease, and cancer.[15] Because milk promotes clogging and mucous formation, it is associated with constipation, especially in children. Some reports suggest that eliminating dairy products from children's diets reduced constipation. If this is a concern among your children, it may be worth a try to eliminate dairy foods for several days.

CONCERNS ABOUT DAIRY PRODUCTS

Another concern with dairy products is that a significant percentage of the world's population is lactose intolerant, meaning they can't digest the milk sugar lactose. We have all been told and grew up believing that milk was a good source of calcium and strengthened bones. The Dairy Council uses celebrities with milk mustaches to promote drinking milk as nutritious and healthy. The Dairy Council even went as far as to promote drinking milk as a beneficial weight-loss measure. These misleading advertisements continued until research proved otherwise and the Dairy Council was forced to remove them.

The idea that drinking milk equates to strong bones is not completely accurate. While an eight-ounce serving of milk provides significant amounts of calcium, approximately 300 milligrams, only about one-third of it is in an absorbable form. Furthermore, the process of pasteurization reduces calcium absorption rates even further. Pasteurization, which the FDA requires, is the process of heating milk or other liquids to a temperature that kills 90 or more percent of bacteria. This potentially leaves 10 percent of the pathogenic bacteria in milk, while destroying the healthy bacteria as well. And recent research suggests that Vitamin D, not milk, is what promotes bone strength.[16] Milk is made up of two protein molecules, casein (which is about 80 percent of milk protein) and whey. Casein is difficult to absorb and is associated with cancer. A Harvard review suggests a positive association between high intake of dairy products and prostate cancer in men, an increase of 50 percent compared to those who consume minimal amounts of dairy products.[17] Whey on the other hand is a high-quality and absorbable complete protein containing all of the essential amino acids.

Another dairy product, cheese, is loaded with salt as a preservative, and Americans love their cheese, putting it on almost anything. Additionally, concerns have been brought forth regarding cheese and casomorphins—natural opiates produced as a part of the casein digestion process. According to Neal Barnard, author of *Breaking the Food Seduction,* natural morphine found in casein causes the production of casomorphins and can lead to addiction.

One dairy product that does have health-promoting effects is yogurt. Yogurt is an excellent source of healthy bacteria, or probiotics. Probiotics inhabit the gut, leaving fewer places for harmful bacteria to latch on to, which helps avoid overgrowth. They have also been associated with improved immune system function and decreased systemic inflammation.[18, 19] The challenge is to find yogurt that isn't loaded with sugar or laced with harmful chemical sweeteners. Most commercially prepared yogurt is overloaded with sugar, almost overcoming the health-promoting benefits of consuming yogurt. It is better to make your own yogurt at home or find a commercial product with reduced sugar or a natural sweetener like honey, stevia, or xylitol.

WHEN MEAT SUSTAINS LIFE

There is wisdom in the last part of verse thirteen. The Lord is directing us to times when it is most acceptable and in fact prudent to consume meat. Before the advent of the refrigerator and freezer, fruits and vegetables could not be stored and kept for long periods. Our forefathers had to eat the fruits and vegetables "in the season thereof" (Doctrine and Covenants 89:11) and could not rely upon a freezer to keep them from spoiling in order to consume them at a later date. Without freezers and refrigerators, they had to rely upon fresh meat to sustain life because it was the only food source available.

When famine occurs, it is generally because crops can't grow. There may be a drought and insufficient rain to produce crops of grain or to grow vegetables or fruits. It may be the result of a natural disaster that destroys crops. When famine occurs, man must seek out whatever food he can obtain. This includes flesh of beasts and fowls of the air, though even animals can be sparse during famines when they too are fighting for scarce resources.

THE BENEFITS OF ABSTAINING FROM MEATS

We have a superb example of the positive health effects of abstaining from meats in the first chapter of Daniel. In this chapter, we read the story of Daniel and other Hebrew children who are brought by Nebuchadnezzar, king of Babylon, into his court to be trained alongside the king's seed and the princes. These were children chosen because they had no blemish and were well favored, wise, skillful, and cunning in knowledge and understanding of science. So we could say that they appear from the description to be healthy both physically and mentally and on equal ground when they were brought into the king's court. As part of this three-year training process, Ashpenaz, the master of the eunuchs, was given charge to supply these children with a portion of the king's meat and wine. However, Daniel knew this was not the most nutritious diet and requested of Ashpenaz that he and other Hebrew children be allowed to eat pulse instead. Pulse is defined as foods made of seeds and grains. Ashpenaz did not want to disobey the king's orders and initially resisted. However, Daniel persuaded him to allow a ten-day trial of the pulse diet versus the traditional diet provided by the king to determine which diet was better. Ashpenaz consented and the trial of diets began. After ten days, those who ate pulse appeared healthier than those who ate the portion of the king's meat and wine.

It is interesting that a noticeable difference could be gained in only ten days. This is another testament to a predominantly plant-based diet. In addition to appearing physically healthier, God blessed Daniel and the other children with "knowledge and skill in all learning and wisdom" (Daniel 1:17). Proper nutrition does appear to correlate with mental capacity and health. Deficiencies in proper foods creates deficiencies in the supply of nutrients to the brain. Foods can and do have a tremendous impact on mood and mental and emotional health. President Ezra Taft Benson said, "There is no question that the health of the body affects the spirit, or the Lord would never have revealed the Word of Wisdom. God has never given any temporal commandments—that which affects our bodies also affects our souls."[20]

THE ENVIRONMENTAL IMPACT OF
MEAT CONSUMPTION

Sparing meat consumption provides obvious enhanced physical health and even mental health, but in addition there are environmental issues important to this subject. The majority of corn and soy grown in the world is used as livestock feed. This is food taken out of the mouths of hungry children and adults in order for the more affluent to gratify their desires for animal flesh. If those accustomed to the westernized diet consumed less meat, there would be less corn and soy required to feed cattle, pigs, and chickens, thus providing more food for the destitute and impoverished. This could make a significant impact in diminishing the 25,000 tragic deaths that occur from starvation and hunger each day.[21] Cattle have stomachs predominantly meant to digest grass. The purpose of feeding cattle grain is to promote rapid weight gain, getting them to market more quickly. The larger the cow, the greater the profits.

There is also the matter of pollution caused by livestock. According to the Environmental Protection Agency, nearly 75 percent of all water quality problems are agriculture related.[22] Much of current agriculture is conducted to feed the animals we consume. Inevitably, animal wastes, hormones, and antibiotics given to livestock get in the water supply. Not too mention the significant amounts of pesticides and chemical fertilizers that are used on crops fed to livestock. If this practice continues unchecked, it is possible the water supply will deteriorate to an unsafe level for human consumption. Large quantities of water are withdrawn for the production of feed and for livestock to drink, again taking this precious resource away from mankind. Livestock play a significant role in greenhouse gas emissions. In fact, the livestock sector generates more greenhouse gas emissions as measured in CO_2 than transportation.[23] Given all the vehicles on this earth, that is an astounding statistic. I would venture to say that the majority of people would believe just the opposite is true. It is estimated that 30 percent of the earths land surface is dedicated to raising livestock, and 70 percent of the former forests of the Amazon have been converted to grazing pastures.[24] This causes significant land degradation and water pollution. Moreover, animals that inhabit the rainforest as well as important plants are destroyed all in the name of satisfying man's desire for meat.

IS VEGETARIANISM THE BEST WAY TO EAT?

This doesn't mean you should abstain completely from meat and become a vegetarian. I am not advocating a strict vegetarian diet at all. The Lord has provided everything on this earth for the use of man, and this includes animals. But we must use prudence and exercise restraint when we consume the flesh of beasts and fowls of the air. Meat in small quantities is part of a healthy diet, but the key is using small quantities of the most healthy meats. I doubt the Lord intended *sparingly* to be two meat meals a day, as is common in affluent societies. According to Merriam-Webster's dictionary, *sparingly* means "marked by or practicing careful restraint (as in the use of resources)." It is beneficial to have several meals per week without any meat included. Instead substitute protein sources such as beans, lentils, soy foods, and whole grains. Reducing meat consumption increases health and benefits the earth.

7

Grains: *The* Staff *of* Life

*All grain is ordained for the use of man and beasts, to be the staff of life,
not only for man but for the beasts of the field, and the fowls of heaven, and all
wild animals that run and creep on the earth; And these hath God made for
use of man only in times of famine and excess hunger. . . . Nevertheless, wheat
for man, and corn for the ox, and oats for the horse, and rye for the fowls and
for swine, and all beasts of the field, and barley for useful animals, and for
mild drinks, as also other grain.*

Doctrine and Covenants 89:14–15, 17

Grains have been cultivated for their edible seed and enjoyed for generations. Grains are the dietary staple of many cultures. Many years ago, our mothers would bake homemade bread—some mothers still do if you are one of the lucky ones. The distinctive and delicious smell of it was obvious upon entering our homes and made our mouths water instantly. Those days are almost entirely gone. Few people take the time to make homemade bread, and if they have time, they probably don't have the knowledge to make it. Instead we consume empty calories from commercially prepared and refined white bread. This unfortunate event is taking a great toll on our health. The grain-refining process removes the bran and germ of grains and takes with it most of the fiber, vitamins and minerals. White flour is produced by refining and often bleaching whole wheat, destroying more than half of the nutrients wheat contains in its whole form. This includes vitamins B1, B2, B3, E, folic acid, calcium, zinc, iron, phosphorus, copper, and fiber. That is a long list of healthful nutrients being destroyed and removed from wheat. Wheat is thus placed in an unnatural, damaged, and less nourishing state—a form less nutrient dense than when God made it and in a state other than how He intended us to eat it. What God has created for man as food cannot be improved by man. In fact, generally when man alters food from its natural state, its nutritional value is reduced. President Benson stated, "the more food we eat in its natural state—the less refined, and the fewer additives it contains—the healthier it will be for us."[1] Not only does homemade whole wheat bread taste and smell better, but it is also healthier.

REFINED VERSUS WHOLE GRAINS

Refined grains are milled and processed to "improve" their appearance and texture, increase their volume, and make them more stable for a longer shelf life. But the outcome of this process is a considerable loss of nutrients. In fact, weevils generally prefer to infest whole-wheat flour versus white flour because white flour provides less nutrients necessary for their survival. If the weevil will die from refined white flour consumption, think about what it is doing to man. This fact reveals that even unintelligent forms of life are able to differentiate between wholesome and unhealthy grains.

Manufacturers have been mandated by governments to attempt to "enrich" refined grains in an effort to overcome the loss of nutrients in processed grains. Using the word *enriched* for this process is erroneous, since the enrichment process only adds vitamins B1, B2, and B3 and iron back to the processed grain. Other essential nutrients such as fiber, calcium, phosphorus, zinc, and folic acid are ignored. Enriching means to improve upon or enhance, and the grain "enriching" process does neither of these as compared to wheat in its whole form.

Grains are called the staff of life because they have been so historically important for mankind's survival and an essential part of our diet for thousands of years. Joseph of Egypt stored grains after interpreting the king of Egypt's dream about seven years of plenty followed by seven lean years (Genesis 41:48-49). Grains store well for many years with minimal nutrient loss, especially when placed in proper containers and stored in a cool dry place at proper temperatures. Whole grains are significant sources of fiber, potassium, iron, the B vitamins, selenium, magnesium, and other essential nutrients.

THE HEALTH BENEFITS OF WHOLE GRAINS

People who eat whole grains instead of refined grains achieve many health benefits, including reduced risk of chronic diseases such as coronary heart disease, atherosclerosis, stroke, obesity, and diabetes.[2] You may be surprised to know that eating whole grains can help you control your weight.[3] Increased consumption of whole grains is inversely associated with weight gain because of its high fiber content, which reduces constipation and water retention. On the other hand, the consumption of refined grains is associated with weight gain. Another factor in weight control is the fact that we usually eat more refined grains because they are not as satisfying as whole grains, thus consuming a greater quantity of empty calories.

Folate gained from whole grains is indispensable during pregnancy to prevent neural tube defects during fetal development. Without proper levels of folate, the developing fetus can experience significant retardation of proper growth. Whole grains also help reduce cholesterol due to their high fiber content. The B vitamins in whole grains play a role in metabolism by helping to release energy from the foods we consume. Magnesium, found in whole grains, helps build strong bones and is a cofactor for enzymes involved in the body's use of glucose and insulin secretion. Selenium, found in whole grains, is a powerful antioxidant, protecting cells from oxidative damage, and helps promote healthy immune system function.

Whole grains contain phytonutrients that act as weak hormone-like substances in the body called lignans. Lignans accelerate the metabolism of estrogen and occupy estrogen receptors in the body, helping to protect against breast cancer in women.[4] In fact premenopausal women that eat greater than thirty grams of fiber per day reduce their risk of breast cancer by 50 percent.[5] Lignans also seem to benefit men because of their ability to bind to and precipitate testosterone, a hormone believed to increase prostate tumor growth.[6] Research suggests that diets rich in lignans are associated with lower incidence of cancer, diabetes, cardio-vascular disease, and kidney disease.[7, 8, 9, 10]

The polyunsaturated fats, plant sterols, saponins, and oligosaccharides in whole grains have cholesterol-lowering effects. High cholesterol is something many Americans suffer with, and eating more whole grains could be of great benefit. You may have seen the many advertisements on oat cereals claiming this effect. Indeed, dietary factors are the most important element of a cholesterol management strategy. A small reduction in cholesterol can provide a significant protective effect against heart disease, the number-one killer of Americans.

Whole grains also have a significant quantity of antioxidants that protect cells against oxidative damage, including selenium and vitamin E. The phytoestrogens in whole grains not only occupy estrogen receptors and bind to testosterone, but they also can affect cholesterol levels and blood vessel elasticity. Thus they promote the health of the cardiovascular system. Clinical trials have indicated that whole grains are associated with increased insulin sensitivity, one of the factors associated with type 2 diabetes.[11] If more whole grains were consumed in the United States, less people would have to suffer with this miserable disease.

Whole grains are complex carbohydrates, meaning that during the digestive process they are broken down in a controlled, regulated manner. This is in contrast to refined carbohydrates that provide a rush of energy because they are broken down so quickly. By metabolizing more slowly, whole grains help prevent a rapid spike in blood sugar, which is associated with an increased risk of diabetes and cardiovascular disease.[12, 13, 14] The bulk of carbohydrates in your diet should be complex. Simple carbohydrates, such as refined sugar and white flour, result in increased caloric intake, and create nutrient deficiencies, as these foods are "empty calories" (high calorie and poor nutrition). When we are full of junk, we are less likely to eat foods with essential nutrients. Complex carbohydrates are also more satisfying as compared to simple carbohydrates, providing a feeling of fullness.

TYPES OF GRAINS

There are many different types of grain, each providing unique flavor, phytonutrients, and health benefits. Worldwide, wheat, corn, and rice make up the majority of grain production. Each culture is different in the type and quantity of grain consumed. In China and India, rice is the favorite grain, while here in the United States and Canada, wheat is the predominant grain. The grains discussed below are the most commonly consumed by man and/or are named in this revelation.

Wheat

The Lord tells us all grains are provided for the use of man and beasts, but He further states that wheat is for man. Wheat is one of the most important crops in the world, providing nourishment for more people than any other food.[15] It appears from the Lord's counsel that we gain more nutritional value and benefit from wheat than any other grain. We may want to consider this the next time we are choosing between whole wheat and white bread. When you compare a slice of white bread with wheat bread, the whole wheat slice has more than fifteen times the amount of vitamin E and three times as much fiber. Among the major grains, wheat has the highest protein content. President Ezra Taft Benson stated, "Most of us are acquainted with some of the prohibitions of the Word of Wisdom. . . . But what needs additional emphasis are the positive aspects—the need for vegetables, fruits, and grain, particularly wheat."[16]

Wheat is full of beneficial nutrients when in its natural and unrefined state, including fiber, manganese, folic acid, calcium phosphorus, zinc, copper, protein, iron, magnesium, and vitamins B1, B2, B3, B5, B6, and E. It is used heavily for breads because of its gluten content. Gluten is a protein found in many grains but in greatest quantities in wheat. It provides elasticity to bread and allows bakers to create satisfying risen bread.

The consumption of whole wheat products is associated with lower incidence of colon cancer and breast cancer, promotes regular bowel function, and reduces the risk of diverticular disease. This information supports the historical use of wheat bran as a bulk laxative. Some of the health benefits of wheat may be due to its metabolite betaine. Betaine has the ability to reduce levels of inflammatory markers that are linked to a number of chronic conditions such as heart disease, diabetes, osteoporosis, and reduced cognitive function. Wheat bran is an anti-cancer food. Interestingly wheat bran has been shown to be beneficial in preventing colon cancer, whereas corn and oats have not shown the same effect.[17] It appears wheat has something extraordinary in it that other grains do not. Another important nutrient in wheat is wheat germ. Wheat germ is a concentrated nutrient source and contains high amounts of oil and vitamin E, which protects the oil from oxidizing too quickly. Vitamin E has healing properties of its own as a powerful antioxidant. Vitamin E helps reduce LDL cholesterol, is an essential nutrient for the immune system, and helps form red blood cells.

Rice

Rice is the second most consumed grain in the world. Over half of the world's population depends on rice for food. It is particularly popular in Asia and India where it is used for most meals. In fact the same word is used for rice and food in China. Unfortunately, just like wheat, most of the rice we consume is in an adulterated form. We seem to prefer white to brown when it comes to our grains. White rice has a more pleasing appearance, is easier for most people to digest, and is less chewy than brown rice. White rice is made by removing the germ and bran of brown rice, stripping it of important nutrients, and then polishing it into white rice. This milling and polishing process removes over 60 percent of the vitamins and minerals contained in brown rice. Brown rice is a good source of protein; vitamins B1, B2, B3, and B6; as well as the minerals phosphorus, iron, selenium, and manganese. In fact, one cup of brown rice supplies almost an entire day's worth of the recommended daily allowance of manganese and over 25 percent of the RDA of selenium. Brown rice is lower in fiber than other grains, but it contains good quantities of essential amino acids. Brown rice is another food that would go a long way in improving the typical westernized diet if it were substituted for the less-nutritious white rice.

Corn

Corn is a versatile grain used both in fresh and dry form. According to the Whole Grains Council, it is the most produced grain worldwide, accounting for 21 percent of human nutrition. It is widely cultivated in America and popular in summer when the ears are ripe. Many farms are covered in the familiar appearance of corn stocks. We even turn these fields into mazes during the fall. Popcorn is low in calories and a popular snack food. You can't watch a movie without popcorn, right? Unfortunately, most corn is not grown for human consumption but rather for livestock consumption or other products such as ethanol fuel, syrups, sweeteners, and oils. Corn provides respectable amounts of vitamins B1, B5, C, and E; folic acid; and the minerals magnesium and phosphorus, as well as good amounts of fiber and essential fatty acids. However, it is not considered a complete food because people who rely heavily upon corn as a food source run the risk of pellagra.[18] Pellagra is a disease caused by a deficiency of niacin. The niacin content in corn is not very absorbable by the intestine unless treated with alkali, as is the case in tortillas. The Native Americans used corn as the staple in their diet but avoided pellagra by adding mineral ash to it when consumed. Corn is also low in protein, but it is a good source of fiber. Corn contains high levels of the antioxidants lycopene and vitamin C, which may slow disease progression. Indeed corn was found to have the greatest antioxidant activity among grains in one study.[19] Yellow corn, the most common corn used today, provides high levels of lutein, a carotenoid linked with protection against heart disease and macular degeneration.[20]

Oats

Oats are the fourth leading grain produced in the United States and famous for their health benefits. Very little of total oat production is consumed by humans since most is fed to livestock. It is predominantly used as a breakfast cereal, like oatmeal. Oatmeal is an excellent and healthy choice for breakfast because it provides sustained energy and helps reduce total and LDL cholesterol.[21] It is digested slowly and methodically rather than quickly like other breakfast cereals. For those who are sensitive to wheat, oat bran is a good substitute. Oat flour can be used in both bread and cookies.

Oats are hulled for consumption, but this does not remove the bran and germ, leaving the nutrients intact. Oats have good quantities of selenium, magnesium, phosphorous, manganese, and iron, as well as fiber and vitamin B1. Oats contain a high percentage of complex carbohydrates, which help reduce the risk of certain cancers, heart disease, diabetes, and bowel irregularity.[22, 23] Oats are famous for their ability to reduce the risk of heart disease, and many cereals manufactured from oats put this claim on their box. Oats also contain an excellent amino acid profile, as well as balanced amounts of essential fatty acids, providing many essential proteins necessary for optimum functioning of the body. Compared to other grains, oats contain high levels of unsaturated fat in the germ. Oats reduce blood glucose and insulin responses, which is essential in preventing diabetes complications. This helps control blood glucose swings associated with diabetes. The polysaccharide in oats, beta-glucan, may enhance immune system function and lower cholesterol levels. Many studies have demonstrated that significant reduction of high cholesterol levels is possible with frequent oat consumption. Oats also contain avenanthramides, antioxidants that help protect the blood vessels from LDL cholesterol damage.

Barley

Barley has a rich flavor similar to nuts and is used as a sweetener as well as to manufacture alcoholic products. Barley is a hardy grain and grows well in cold climates. Most barley is fed to livestock. Barley has a similar nutritional makeup to corn, but it contains good quantities of niacin and high levels of fiber and selenium. Barley's fiber is found throughout the grain, which may be the reason it has the highest fiber content of any grain. The fiber in barley, like oats, is high in beta-glucan, which helps lower cholesterol and reduces the risk of heart disease. Barley drinks have been used medicinally for many years, and some research suggests that these drinks may help prevent diabetes by increasing insulin sensitivity.[24]

Rye

Rye has an appearance similar to that of wheat. It is hardy, growing in inhospitable soil and cold climates. Rye can be used without other grains to produce pleasing leavened bread. Bread produced from rye is more dense and heavier than bread produced from wheat. It has a lower glycemic index than most grains and is therefore beneficial to diabetics. The type of fiber in rye promotes a prompt feeling of fullness, making it an ideal grain to consume when trying to lose weight. Rye is an excellent source of manganese and selenium and provides good levels of phosphorous, magnesium, and protein. In 2007, scientists discovered that a rye diet can modify gene expression.[25] This is important for those who feel it is inevitable that they will have a certain disease because of the genes they inherited.

8

Benefits *and* Blessings

And all saints who remember to keep and do these sayings, walking in obedience to the commandments, shall receive health in their navel and marrow in their bones; And shall find wisdom and great treasures of knowledge, even hidden treasures; And shall run and not be weary, and shall walk and not faint. And I, the Lord, give them a promise, that the destroying angel shall pass by them, as the children of Israel, and not slay them. Amen.

Doctrine and Covenants 89:18–21

God wants us to have joy and happiness. One of the conditions for us to realize this joy and happiness is obedience to His law of health. Members of The Church of Jesus Christ of Latter-day Saints commit to following the Word of Wisdom, which entails so much more than abstaining from tea and coffee. The Word of Wisdom includes avoidance of all harmful substances, but more importantly teaches us that which is beneficial and nourishing to the body. Obedience to the Word of Wisdom is a matter of personal worthiness for members of the Church. After all, blessings are predicated on obedience, and obedience means we are willing to submit our will to the Father's. The Lord created and gave us miraculous physical bodies, and He expects us to take proper care of them. Those who live the Word of Wisdom to its fullest will generally live longer and more worthwhile lives. President Gordon B. Hinckley said, "I give thanks to our Creator for revealing unto His prophet what we call the Word of Wisdom. I do not hesitate to say that in this brief but inclusive statement of the Lord is found counsel, given with a promise, which, if more widely observed, would save untold pain and suffering and lead not only to increased physical well-being but also to great and satisfying 'treasures of knowledge' of the things of God."[1]

THE FAR-REACHING BENEFITS OF
THE WORD OF WISDOM

There is too much disease and premature death and too few healthy people in the world today. The Word of Wisdom has never been needed more than it is now. Obedience to this revelation will bring greater health and vitality and ultimately a greater quality of life, not just quantity. This doesn't mean that you will be disease free or avoid death. It means you will achieve your personal level of optimum health. You will be able to live your life to the fullest, gaining the fullest experiences necessary for you to progress in God's eternal plan. Your body will be fortified with a greater resistance to disease and illness, and your immune system will be stronger. However, don't be discouraged if you experience disease and ill health despite living the Word of Wisdom. Everything that happens to us happens for a purpose and is part of God's plan. You may need to experience ill health and adversity to become what He wants you to become. And death and disease are both part of mortal life. Death is a necessary step toward the next realm of existence, and disease is often necessary to strengthen and try us. If we never experience sickness and pain, we will not fully appreciate health and pleasure.

With better health comes a realized decrease in health expenditures. As you take care of your body and avoid harmful substances, you will spend less on "sick" care and prevent wasteful expenditures on harmful substances. Imagine what you could save if you stop filling your thirty-two-ounce mug twice or more daily with soda and replace it with water. The savings of someone who currently smokes goes beyond just the cost of a pack of cigarettes. The health care savings of quitting smoking will be immeasurable in the long run. Additionally, if you abstain from smoking in the first place you will preclude yourself from enduring the difficult process of overcoming addiction. Addiction is challenging and problematic to overcome. It requires a strong conviction and desire to quit, coupled with the support of family, friends, health professionals, and wise leaders. If you have already succumbed to addiction, I urge you to begin now the process back to physical and spiritual health. As you eliminate and overcome your addiction, you will see measurable improvements in your health and well being. The process of overcoming addiction will be challenging, and you will face many struggles, but it will be well worth it. You will replace temporary pleasure with true and long-term joy. You may not be successful at first, but you can beat the addiction if you have the desire to do so and receive the necessary help. Don't forget to plead for help from the Lord. And definitely don't feel unworthy to speak to Him. He is anxious to help you. He waits with open arms and outstretched hands, willing to listen to you and give you all the help you need. He will not leave you alone to complete this task if you ask for His help.

The Word of Wisdom is not just for the physical body. Obedience to the Word of Wisdom also promises increased wisdom, knowledge, and spiritual power. Disobedience to it will result in damage to spiritual growth and a decreased capacity to avoid other detrimental practices. Wisdom is the proper use of knowledge. The Word of Wisdom provides knowledge, and those who live its precepts are exercising wisdom. President Joseph Fielding Smith said, "The truth is that spiritual salvation is dependent upon the temporal far more than most men realize. The line of demarcation between the temporal, or physical, and the spiritual, cannot be definitely seen. The Lord has said that he has not given a temporal commandment at any time. To men some of these commandments may be temporal, but they are spiritual to the Lord because they all have a bearing on the spiritual, or eternal welfare of mankind."[2] It is obvious that how we treat the physical body directly correlates with our spiritual health. When we have an active, healthy body, our inner spiritual strength can grow and thrive. Optimum physical health affords maximum mental capacity. We have a greater capacity to learn and think clearly when our physical bodies are healthy. With this greater capacity will come the "wisdom and great treasures of knowledge, even hidden treasures" the Lord promises (Doctrine and Covenants 89:19).

THE WORD OF WISDOM IS THE FOUNDATION, BUT PERSONAL REVELATION IS NECESSARY

The Word of Wisdom is simple and practical but does not spell out everything we should and should not consume. The Lord will not "command in all things" (Doctrine and Covenants 58:26) nor provide a detailed list for us to follow. The Lord expects us to use prudence and wisdom and exercise personal judgment based upon the guidance in this revelation. Again quoting President Joseph Fielding Smith, "Such revelation is unnecessary. The Word of Wisdom is a basic law. It points the way and gives us ample instruction in regard to both food and drink, good for the body and also detrimental. If we sincerely follow what is written with the aid of the Spirit of the Lord, we need no further counsel. . . . Thus by keeping the commandments we are promised inspiration and the guidance of the Spirit of the Lord through which we will know what is good and what is bad for the body."[3] Prayerful and thoughtful consideration is necessary because each one of us has different needs. We are all biologically different. As we follow the Lord's counsel and seek personal inspiration, the Lord will guide us to the best foods for us individually and for our families.

SCIENTIFIC SUPPORT OF THE WORD OF WISDOM— LONGER LIFE AND LESS CANCER

While the Word of Wisdom does not need scientific evidence to back it up, much of current scientific research lends credence to its principles and truthfulness. Looking at life expectancy for members of The Church of Jesus Christ of Latter-day Saints in Utah compared to non-members reveals a greater life expectancy. Male members of the Church live an average of 7.3 years longer than non-member men and women live an average of 5.8 years longer than non-member women.[4] Cancer research also supports the Word of Wisdom. Male and female members of the Church have a 24 percent lower incidence of all cancers as compared to non-members living in Utah.[4] It appears proper dietary habits are more important than location.

DISCOVER THE BLESSINGS OF
THE WORD OF WISDOM FOR YOURSELF

I testify that the Word of Wisdom was given to the Prophet Joseph Smith directly from the Lord. It is meant for our benefit, for us to gain the best health and well-being possible. Obedience to the counsel contained therein will bring blessings to those who follow it—both temporal and spiritual. With obedience to the principles it contains, greater physical health, more self-control, greater clarity of mind, and more spiritual power will be realized. You will gain a closer relationship with your Heavenly Father and His Son, Jesus Christ. I urge all of us to carefully examine what we take into our bodies and make the necessary changes to gain all the blessings and rewards our Father in Heaven is waiting anxiously to provide.

Appendix A

Fruit and Vegetable Nutrient Content

FRUITS

Fruit	Vitamins	Minerals	Phytonutrients & Other Nutrients
Apple (raw with skin, 1 cup, quartered)	Folate (4 mcg) Vitamin A (68 IU) Vitamin C (5.7 mg) Vitamin E (.23 mg)	Calcium (7 mg) Potassium (134 mg) Phosphorus (14 mg) Magnesium (6 mg)	Fiber (2.9 mg) Pectin Quercetin
Apricot (raw, 1 cup, halved)	Vitamin A (2985 IU) Vitamin C (15.5 mg)	Calcium (21 mg) Iron (.6 mg) Potassium (402 mg)	Beta-carotene (1695 mcg) Lutein Protein (2.17 g) Quercetin

Avocado (raw, 1 cup, cubed)	Folate (122 mcg) Niacin (2.6 mg) Pantothenic Acid (2.1 mg) Vitamin A (219 IU) Vitamin B1 (.1 mg) Vitamin B2 (.2 mg) Vitamin B6 (.39 mg) Vitamin C (15 mg)	Calcium (18 mg) Iron (.82 mg) Magnesium (43 mg) Phosphorus (79 mg) Potassium (728 mg) Sodium (10 mg)	Alpha-carotene (36.09 mcg) Beta-carotene (92.37 mcg) Cryptoxanthin Fiber (10 g) Lutein Protein (2.99 g) Quercetin
Banana (raw, 1 cup, sliced)	Folate (30 mcg) Niacin (1 mg) Pantothenic Acid (.5 mg) Vitamin A (96 IU) Vitamin B6 (.55 mg) Vitamin C (13.1 mg) Vitamin E (.15 mg)	Calcium (8 mg) Iron (.38 mg) Magnesium phosphorus (32 mg) Potassium (537 mg) Selenium (1.5 mcg)	Alpha-carotene (39.05 mcg) Beta-carotene (37.41 mcg) Fiber (5.7 g) Lutein Protein (1.64 g) Rutin
Blackberry (raw, 1 cup)	Folate (9 mcg) Vitamin A (80 IU) Vitamin C (14.4 mg) Vitamin E (.84 mg)	Calcium Iron (.41 mg) Magnesium (9 mg) Manganese (.08 mg) Phosphorus (18 mg) Potassium (114 mg) Selenium (.2 mcg) Zinc (.23 mg)	Epicatechin Fiber (3.6 g) Protein (2.0 g) Quercetin
Cantaloupe (raw, 1 cup, balls)	Folate (38 mcg) Vitamin A (5985 IU) Vitamin B6 (.13 mg) Vitamin C (65 mg)	Calcium (17 mg) Magnesium (21 mg) Phosphorus (27 mg) Potassium (473 mg)	Beta-carotene (3575.74 IU) Fiber (1.6 g) Protein (1.48 g) Rutin

Cherry (sweet, raw, 1 cup, without pits)	Vitamin A (98 IU) Vitamin C (10.8 mg)	Calcium (20 mg) Copper (.08 mg) Iron (.55 mg) Magnesium (17 mg) Manganese (.11 mg) Phosphorus (33 mg) Potassium (341 mg)	Anthocyanins Epicatechin
Cranberry (raw, 1 cup, whole)	Vitamin A (60 IU) Vitamin C (13.3 mg)	Calcium (8 mg) Phosphorus (13 mg) Potassium (85 mg) Selenium (.1 mcg)	Catechin Epicatechin Quercetin
Grape (raw, red or green, seedless, 1 cup)	Folate (3 mcg) Niacin (.28 mg) Vitamin A (100 IU) Vitamin C (16.3 mg)	Calcium (16 mg) Magnesium (11 mg) Phosphorus (31 mg) Potassium (289 mg)	Beta-carotene (59.52 mg) Protein (1.08 g) Resveratrol Saponins Quercetin
Grapefruit (raw, white, 1 cup, sections, with juice)	Vitamin C (76.6 mg) Vitamin A (75 IU)	Calcium (28 mg) Magnesium (21 mg) Phosphorus (18 mg) Potassium (340 mg)	Fiber (2.5 g) Limanoids Lycopene Pectin Protein (1.59 g)
Kiwi (raw, 1 cup)	Folate (44 mcg) Niacin (.6 mg) Vitamin A (154 IU) Vitamin B2 (.05 mg) Vitamin B6 (.11 mg) Vitamin C (164.1 mg) Vitamin E (2.58 mg)	Calcium (60 mg) Copper (.23 mg) Iron (.55 mg) Magnesium (29 mg) Phosphorus (60 mg) Potassium (552 mg) Selenium (.4 mcg) Zinc (.24 mg)	Beta-carotene (92.83 mg) Cryptoxanthin Fiber (5.4 g) Lutein Protein (2.02 g) Quercetin Zeaxanthin

Lemon (raw, without peel, 1 cup)	Vitamin A (48 IU) Vitamin C (112.4 mg)	Calcium (55 mg) Iron (1.27 mg) Magnesium (17 mg) Phosphorus (34 mg) Potassium (293 mg)	Coumarins Fiber (5.9 g) Limonene Protein (2.33 g)
Lime (raw, one fruit)	Folate (5 mg) Vitamin A (33 IU) Vitamin C (19.5 mg)	Calcium (22 mg) Iron (.4 mg) Magnesium (4 mg) Phosphorus (12 mg) Potassium (68 mg)	Coumarins Fiber (1.9 g)
Mango (raw, 1 cup, sliced)	Folate (23 mg) Niacin (.96 mg) Vitamin A (1262 IU) Vitamin B2 (.09 mg) Vitamin B6 (.22 mg) Vitamin C (45.7 mg) Vitamin E (1.85 mg)	Calcium (17 mg) Magnesium (15 mg) Phosphorus (18 mg) Potassium (257 mg) Selenium (1 mcg)	Catechin Fiber (3.0 g) Limonene Quercetin
Olive (raw, 1 cup, ripe, canned, small to extra large)	Vitamin A (544 IU) Vitamin E (2.24 mg)	Calcium (112 mg) Iron (4.48 mg) Selenium (1.6 mcg) Sodium (1168 mg)	Beta-carotene (3792 IU) Cryptoxanthin
Orange (raw, 1 cup, sections)	Folate (55 mg) Pantothenic Acid (.45 mg) Vitamin A (404 IU) Vitamin B1 (.16 mg) Vitamin C (95.8 mg)	Calcium (72 mg) Magnesium (18 mg) Phosphorus (25 mg) Potassium (326 mg) Selenium (.9 mcg)	Beta-carotene (127.93 IU) Fiber (4.3 g) Hesperidin Limonene Protein (1.69 g) Quercetin

Peach (raw, 1 cup, slices)	Folate (5 mg) Niacin (1.24 mg) Vitamin A (501 IU) Vitamin C (10.2 mg)	Calcium (9 mg) Magnesium (13 mg) Phosphorus (31 mg) Potassium (293 mg) Selenium (.1 mg)	Catechin Fiber (2.3 g) Protein (1.41 g) Quercetin
Pear (raw, 1 small fruit)	Folate (11 mg) Vitamin A (34 IU) Vitamin C (6.2 mg)	Calcium (14 mg) Manganese (.07 mg) Potassium (176 mg) Selenium (.1 mcg)	Fiber (4.5 g) Catechin Epicatechin Quercetin
Pineapple (raw, 1 cup, chunks, tradi-tional variety)	Folate (17 mg) Niacin (.78 mg) Vitamin A (86 IU) Vitamin C (27.9 mg)	Calcium (21 mg) Magnesium (21 mg) Manganese (2.63 mg) Potassium (206 mg) Selenium (.1 mcg)	Beta-carotene (51.56 IU) Bromelain Fiber (2.3 g)
Plum (raw, 1 cup, sliced)	Vitamin A (570 IU) Vitamin C (15.7 mg)	Calcium (10 mg) Potassium (258 mg)	Catechin Epicatechin Fiber (2.3 g) Protein (1.16 g) Quercetin
Raspberry (raw, 1 cup)	Folate (26 mg) Niacin (.74 mg) Vitamin C (32.2 mg)	Calcium (31 mg) Iron (.85 mg) Magnesium (27 mg) Potassium (186 mg)	Fiber (8.0 g) Protein (1.47 g) Quercetin Selenium (.3 mcg)
Strawberry (raw, 1 cup, halves)	Folate (37 mg) Vitamin A (18 IU) Vitamin C (89.3 mg)	Calcium Magnesium (19 mg) Phosphorus (37 mg) Potassium (233 mg) Selenium (.6 mcg)	Fiber Fiber (3 g) Protein (1.01 g) Quercetin

Watermelon (raw, 1 cup, balls)	Folate (4 mg) Niacin (.28 mg) Vitamin A (877 IU) Vitamin B1 (.05 mg) Vitamin B6 (.07 mg) Vitamin C (12.5 mg)	Calcium (11 mg) Iron (.36 mg) Magnesium (15 mg) Phosphorus (18 mg) Potassium (173 mg) Selenium (.6 mg)	Beta-carotene (466.39 mg) Lutein Lycopene

VEGETABLES

Vegetable	Vitamins	Minerals	Phytonutrients & Other Nutrients
Beet (cooked, boiled, drained, sliced, no salt, 1 cup)	Folate (136 mg) Niacin (.56 mg) Vitamin A (58 mg)	Calcium (28 mg) Copper (.13 mg) Iron (1.34 mg) Magnesium (40 mg) Manganese (.55 mg) Phosphorus (64 mg) Potassium (518 mg)	Fiber (1.7 g) Protein (1.43 g) Quercetin
Broccoli (cooked, boiled, drained, no salt, small stalk— about 5" long)	Folate (151 mg) Vitamin A (2167 IU) Vitamin C (90.9 mg)	Calcium (56 mg) Iron (.94 mg) Magnesium (29 mg) Phosphorus (94 mg) Potassium (410 mg)	Fiber (4.7 g) Lutein Protein (3.33 g) Zeaxanthin
Cabbage (cooked, boiled, drained, no salt, 100 grams of edible portion)	Folate (22 mg) Vitamin C (1.7 mg)	Selenium (1.0 mcg)	Chlorophyll Lutein Quercetin

Carrot (baby, raw, 85 g)	Vitamin A (586 IU) Vitamin C (2.2 mg)	Calcium (27 mg) Iron (.76 mg) Magnesium (9 mg) Selenium (.7 mg)	Alpha-carotene (3201.53 IU) Beta-carotene (5432.35 IU) Coumarins Fiber (2.5 g) Lutein Lycopene Quercetin
Cauliflower (cooked, boiled, drained, without salt, 1 cup)	Folate (54 mg) Vitamin C (55 mg)	Calcium (20 mg) Magnesium (12 mg) Potassium (176 mg) Selenium (.8 mcg)	Beta-sitosterol Fiber (2.8 g) Protein (2.28 g) Quercetin
Celery (raw, 1 cup, chopped)	Folate (36 mg) Vitamin A (454 IU) Vitamin C (3.1 mg)	Calcium (41 mg) Iodine Iron (.2 mg) Magnesium (11 mg) Potassium (263 mg) Zinc (.13 mg)	Coumarins Fiber (1.6 g) Quercetin Rutin
Corn (sweet, yellow, boiled, drained, no salt, 1 medium ear— about 7" long)	Folate (48 mg) Niacin (1.66 mg) Vitamin A (271 mg)	Magnesium (27 mg) Phosphorus (77 mg) Potassium (219 mg) Selenium (.2 mg)	Beta-carotene (67.82 IU) Fiber (2.9 g) Protein (3.42 g)
Cucumber (raw, peeled, sliced, 1 cup)	Folate (17 mg) Vitamin A (86 IU) Vitamin C (3.8 mg)	Calcium (17 mg) Iron (.27 mg) Magnesium(14 mg) Potassium (162 mg)	Beta-carotene (36.44 mg) Beta-sitosterol

Green Beans (raw, snapped, 1 cup)	Folate (22 mg) Vitamin A (71 IU) Vitamin K (6.8 mcg)	Calcium (18 mg) Iron (.61 mg) Magnesium (9 mg) Selenium (.3 mcg)	Beta-carotene (63 IU)
Lettuce (green leaf, raw, 2 cups, shredded)	Folate (28 mg) Vitamin A (5332 IU) Vitamin C (13 mg)	Calcium (26 mg) Iron (.62 mg) Potassium (140 mg) Selenium (.4 mcg)	Chlorophyll Fiber (1 g) Lutein Pectin
Onion (raw, sliced, 1 cup)	Folate (21 mg) Vitamin C (8.5 mg)	Calcium (26 mg) Iron (.24 mg) Magnesium (11 mg) Selenium (.5 mg) Zinc (.19 mg)	Fiber (2.0 g) Protein (1.26 g) Quercetin Rutin Saponins
Pea (green, cooked, boiled, drained, no salt, 1 cup)	Folate (101 mg) Vitamin A (1282 IU) Vitamin C (22.7 mg) Vitamin E (.22 mg)	Calcium (43 mg) Iron (2.46 mg) Magnesium (62 mg) Phosphorus (187 mg) Potassium (434 mg)	Alpha-carotene (35.44 IU) Beta-carotene (751.42 IU) Fiber (8.8 mg) Lutein Protein (8.58 mg)
Pepper (sweet, green, raw, sliced, 1 cup)	Folate (10 mg) Niacin (.44 mg) Vitamin A (340 IU) Vitamin C (74 mg)	Calcium (9 mg) Iron (.31 mg) Potassium (261 mg)	Alpha-carotene (18.9 IU) Beta-carotene (191.73 IU) Bioflavonoids Fiber (1.5 g) Lutein Quercetin

Potato (baked, with skin, no salt, 1 medium)	Folate (48 mg) Niacin (2.44 mg) Pantothenic Acid (.65 mg) Vitamin B1 (.11 mg) Vitamin C (16.6 mg)	Calcium (26 mg) Iron (1.88 mg) Magnesium (49 mg) Manganese (.38 mg) Phosphorus (120 mg) Potassium (925 mg) Zinc (.61 mg)	Fiber (3.8 g) Lutein Protein (4.32 g) Quercetin Rutin
Pumpkin (pie mix, canned, 1 cup)	Niacin (1.01 mg) Pantothenic Acid (3.07 mg) Vitamin A (22405 IU) Vitamin C (9.5 mg)	Calcium (100 mg) Iron (2.86 mg) Magnesium (43 mg) Phosphorus (122 mg) Potassium (373 mg) Sodium (562 mg)	Beta-carotene Cryptoxanthin Fiber (22.4 g) Lutein Protein (2.94 g) Quercetin Zeaxanthin
Radish (raw, slices, 1 cup)	Folate (28 mg) Vitamin C (17.2 mg)	Calcium (29 mg) Iron (.39 mg) Selenium (.7 mg) Zinc (.33 mcg)	Fiber (1.9 g)
Spinach (raw, 2 cups)	Folate (116 mg) Niacin (.43 mg) Vitamin A (5626 IU) Vitamin C (16.8 mg)	Calcium (60 mg) Copper (.08 mg) Iron (1.6 mg) Magnesium (48 mg) Manganese (.54 mg) Potassium (334 mg) Zinc (.32 mg)	Beta-carotene (3375.8 IU) Fiber (1.4 g) Lutein Protein (1.72 g) Zeaxanthin
Squash (summer, all varieties, cooked, boiled, drained, no salt, 1 cup, slices)	Folate (36 mg) Vitamin A (381 IU) Vitamin C (9.9 mg)	Calcium (49 mg) Iron (.65 mg) Magnesium (43 mg) Phosphorus (70 mg) Potassium (346 mg) Selenium (.4 mcg)	Beta-carotene (228.61 IU) Fiber (2.5 g) Pectin Protein (1.64 g)

Sweet Potato (cooked, baked in skin, without salt, 1 medium—5" long)	Niacin (1.7 mg) Pantothenic Acid (1 mg) Vitamin A (21909 IU) Vitamin C (22.3 mg)	Calcium (43 mg) Iron (.79 mg) Potassium (542 mg) Selenium (.2 mcg) Zinc (.36 mg)	Alpha-carotene (49.5 IU) Beta-carotene (13120.65 IU) Fiber (3.8 g) Pectin Protein (2.29 g)
Tomato (red, ripe, raw, year-round average, 1 cup, chopped or sliced)	Folate (27 mg) Niacin (1.07 mg) Vitamin A (1500 IU) Vitamin B6 (.14 mg) Vitamin C (22.8 mg)	Calcium (18 mg) Iron (.49 mg) Magnesium (20 mg) Phosphorus (43 mg) Potassium (426 mg) Sodium (8 mg)	Beta-carotene (808.85 IU) Fiber (2.2 g) Lycopene Protein (1.59 g) Quercetin
Yam (cooked, boiled or baked, no salt, 1 cup, cubes)	Folate (22 mg) Vitamin A (165 IU) Vitamin C (16.5 mg)	Calcium (19 mg) Iron (.71 mg) Magnesium (24 mg) Potassium (911 mg) Selenium (1.0 mcg)	Fiber (5.3 g) Protein (2.03 g)

Appendix B

Vitamins, Minerals, *and* Other Nutrients

Vitamin/Mineral	**DRI** (Dietary Reference Intake)	Function/Purpose
Vitamin A	3000 IU	✓ Helps maintain hair, bones, and teeth ✓ Essential for eyes and skin ✓ Promotes proper immune system function
Vitamin B1 (Thiamin)	1.2 mg	✓ Necessary for carbohydrate metabolism ✓ Necessary for muscle coordination ✓ Promotes healthy nerve function

Vitamin B2 (Riboflavin)	1.8 mg	✓ Necessary for food metabolism and the energy gained from food ✓ Makes Vitamin B6 active in the body ✓ Beneficial for proper tissue repair
Vitamin B3 (Niacin)	16 mg	✓ Necessary to obtain energy from food ✓ Helps break down and use energy from carbohydrates, proteins, and fats ✓ Promotes healthy nerve function ✓ Promotes proper gastrointestinal system function ✓ Helps maintain healthy skin
Vitamin B5 (Pantothenic Acid)	5 mg	✓ Helps the glands produce hormones and chemicals that regulate nerve function ✓ Helps create new fats and proteins in the body
Vitamin B6 (Pyridoxine)	1.7 mg	✓ Necessary for protein metabolism and absorption ✓ Necessary for carbohydrate metabolism ✓ Promotes nerve and brain function ✓ Plays a role in many enzymatic reactions within the body

Vitamin B12 (Cyano-cobalamin)	2 mcg	✓ Promotes normal nerve function ✓ Promotes normal blood function ✓ Helps form red blood cells
Folate (Folic Acid)	400 mg	✓ Helps prevent birth defects during pregnancy ✓ Essential for red blood cell formation ✓ Essential for protein metabolism
Vitamin C	90 mg	✓ Helps prevent oxidative damage ✓ Helps bind cells together ✓ Helps strengthen blood vessels ✓ Aids in the absorption of iron and copper ✓ Helps form collagen ✓ Helps regenerate and stabilize other vitamins ✓ Important for proper growth and repair of all body tissues ✓ Beneficial to the immune system
Vitamin D	400 IU	✓ Helps absorb calcium and phosphorus ✓ Helps build and maintain strong teeth and bones

Vitamin E	15 mg	✓ Helps prevent oxidative damage
		✓ Helps form red blood cells
		✓ Helps form muscles and other tissues
		✓ Beneficial to the immune system
Vitamin K	120 mcg	✓ Necessary for normal blood clotting
Calcium	1300 mg	✓ Necessary for the development and maintenance of bones and teeth
		✓ Promotes muscle and nerve function
		✓ Helps activate enzymes necessary to convert food to energy
		✓ Beneficial to cardiovascular health
		✓ Helps blood clotting
Copper	.9 mg	✓ Helps several enzymes function properly
		✓ Helps form connective tissue
		✓ Helps iron absorption
		✓ Necessary to form red blood cells
		✓ Important in the production of collagen, cartilage, bone, and connective tissue

Iron	18 mg	✓ Essential to form hemoglobin (the substance in blood that carries oxygen to the cells of the body)
Magnesium	420 mg	✓ Activates enzymes needed to release energy in the body
		✓ Helps regulate potassium levels
		✓ Essential for healthy bones and teeth
		✓ Helps the muscles relax
Manganese	2.3 mg	✓ Essential for healthy bones and cartilage
		✓ Necessary for normal tendon structure
		✓ Helps facilitate metabolism of carbohydrates, fats, and protein
Phosphorus	1250 mg	✓ Helps build bones and teeth
		✓ Necessary for metabolism of fats, proteins, and carbohydrates
		✓ Helps maintain proper urine and blood acid/base balance
Potassium	N/A	✓ Helps the muscles contract
		✓ Helps maintain regular fluid balance
		✓ Necessary for nerve and muscle function

Selenium	55 mcg	✓ Helps prevent oxidative damage
Sodium	N/A	✓ Helps maintain water balance throughout the body ✓ Essential for nerve impulses
Zinc	11 mg	✓ Essential for normal growth and development ✓ Beneficial to the immune system ✓ Necessary for many enzymatic reactions that aid digestion and metabolism ✓ Stimulates wound and burn healing

Bromelain is an anti-inflammatory, proteolytic enzyme from pineapples. It aids the body in the digestion of protein, can help break down mucus in respiratory conditions, and is a potent anti-inflammatory agent.

Beta-sitosterol is a phytosterol (plant compound similar to cholesterol and steroid hormones). It limits cholesterol absorption within the body by blocking absorption sites. It has also been studied for its immune-enhancing effects as well as for its anti-cancer properties.[1]

Carotenoids (alpha-carotene, beta-carotene, cryptoxanthin, lycopene, zeaxanthin, astaxanthin, and lutein) are the source of orange, yellow, and red colors in plants. They are potent antioxidants, meaning they help prevent oxidation of cells. Alpha-carotene, beta-carotene, and beta-cryptoxanthin convert to retinol (vitamin A) in the body without the risk of toxicity. The conversion of these carotenoids to retinol decreases when the body's stores of vitamin A are high. The antioxidant ability of carotenoids has been associated with decreased risk of certain cancers.[2]

Chlorophyll is plants' primary mechanism of photosynthesis (the process of transforming sunlight into fuel for cells). It gives plants their green color and is known as the plants' "blood." The list of health-promoting benefits from chlorophyll is long. It provides nourishment to the intestines, soothes the mucous linings, and detoxifies and purifies the body.[3] In addition, it has antioxidant, anti-inflammatory, and wound-healing properties and removes carbon dioxide and carbon monoxide from the body.

Coumarins are suspected of blocking the carcinogenic effects of chemicals and toxins. They have antitumor properties and stimulate the immune system and the enzyme responsible for anti-carcinogenic properties.

Flavonoids (anthocyanin, bioflavonoids, catechin, epicatechin, hesperidin, quercetin, and rutin) are antioxidant nutrients that provide color and flavor to the plants. These plant compounds provide protective benefits to plants, such as repairing damage and shielding the plant from toxins. Flavonoids are in large supply in fruits and vegetables. There are a large number of flavonoids, each of which provides its own list of health benefits, including antitumor, immune-enhancing, and antioxidant effects. Flavonoids work synergistically with and increase the effectiveness and absorption of vitamin C.

Fiber plays the important role of speeding the body's elimination process. Insoluble fiber, found in many whole grains, is indigestible, adding bulk to digestive materials and speeding its movement through the digestive tract. This prevents toxins that have been sent for elimination from staying in the body, reducing the risk of disease and gallstones. Soluble fiber, found in fruits, vegetables, beans, legumes, seeds, oats, and barley, helps eliminate cholesterol and bile acids, which provides a protective benefit to the cardiovascular system. Adequate intake of fiber reduces constipation and can help prevent diverticular disease.

Limanoids exert antifungal, anticancer, antiviral, and bactericidal effects. They have shown the ability to prevent the initiation of cancer and prevent the growth of certain tumors and cancers.[4]

Pectin, a soluble fiber mostly found in apples and citrus fruits, has the potential to lower cholesterol, improves insulin response, relieves diarrhea, and stimulates the immune system. Pectin promotes a feeling of fullness, possibly reducing overeating.

Resveratrol inhibits the initiation, promotion, and progression of cancer. It is a superb antioxidant and promotes cardiovascular health by lowering LDL cholesterol and reducing plaque buildup in the arteries.

Proteins are an important part of cell function and are the building blocks of any living organism. Proteins are utilized to make enzymes, hormones, and other body chemicals and are necessary for healthy nails and hair, as well as to build and repair tissues. Protein are essential for growth and maintenance.

Saponins are predominantly found in legumes and soy products. They bind to cholesterol, helping to remove it from the body. In addition they may exert anticancer and anti-inflammatory properties. Saponins can also boost immune system activity, particularly the activity of interferon and T-lymphocytes. Research has indicated antitumor properties and the ability to kill cancer cells.[5]

Notes

INTRODUCTION

1. S. Skeel, "What if no one were fat?" accessed April 30, 2008, www. articles.moneycentral.msn.com/Insurance/Advice?WhatIfNoOneWereFat .aspx?.

2. Gordon B. Hinckley, "Joseph Smith Jr.—Prophet of God, Mighty Servant," *Ensign* (December 2005), 2–6.

CHAPTER 1

1. American Institute for Cancer Research, "Food, Nutrition, and the Prevention of Cancer: A Global Perspective" (World Cancer Research Fund: American Institute for Cancer Research, 1997), accessed April 3, 2008, www. aicr.org/publications/cancer-resource/cancerresource_introduction.html.

2. Center for Disease Control, "Leading Causes of Death," accessed April 3, 2008, www.cdc.gov/nchs/faststats/lcod.htm.

3. H. C. Hung, et al, "Deaths: Final Data for 2005: National Vital Statistics Reports" (National Center for Health Statistics, 2008).

4. Ashima K. Kant, Barry I. Graubard, and Arthur Schatzkin, "Dietary Patterns Predict Mortality in National Cohort: The National Health Interview Surveys, 1987 and 1992," *Journal of Nutrition* 134 (2004): 1793–99.

5. T. C. Campbell and T. M. Campbell, *The China Study* (Dallas: Benbella Books, 2004), 24.

6.   Lara J. Akinbami, "The State of Childhood Asthma, United States, 1980–2005," in *Advance Data from Vital and Health Statistics* 381 (December 2006), 3, accessed April 8, 2008, www.cdc.gov/hchs/data/ad/ad381.pdf.

7.   M. Karvonen, J. Pitkanieni, and J. Tuomilehto, "The Onset Age of Type 1 Diabetes in Finnish Children Has Become Younger," *Diabetes Care* 22 (July 1999), 1066–70.

8.   E. J. Schoenle et al. "Epidemiology of Type 1 Diabetes Mellitus in Switzerland: Steep Rise in Incidence in Under 5 Year Old Children in the Past Decade," *Diabetologica* 44 (March 2001), 286–89.

9.   Associated Press, "Skip the Whole Milk. Pass on Soda. Drink Beer?" last modified March 8, 2006, http://www.msnbc.msn.com/id/11735125/ns/health-fitness/t/skip-whole-milk-pass-soda-drink-beer/#.UJqro4V0HyU.

10.   Lenard I. Lesser et al., "Relationship between Funding Source and Conclusion among Nutrition-Related Scientific Articles," *PLoS Medicine* 4(1): e5.

11.   N. Rigotti et al., "Interventions for smoking cessation in hospitalised patients," Cochrane Database System Review, 2007.

12.   P. A. Diethelm, J. C. Rielle, and M. McKee, "The Whole Truth and Nothing but the Truth? The Research Phillip Morris Did Not Want You to See," *Lancet* 364, no. 9446 (July 2005): 86–92.

13.   Joseph Fielding Smith, Conference Report, October 1913, 14.

14.   Center for Disease Control, "Alcohol-Attributable Deaths and Years of Potential Life Lost—United States, 2001," accessed April 16, 2008, www.cdc.gov/MMWR/preview/mmwrhtml/mm5337a2.htm#tab.

15.   Ibid.

CHAPTER 2

1.   S. Arranz et al., "Wine, Beer, Alcohol and Polyphenols on Cardiovascular Disease and Cancer," *Nutrients* 4, no. 7 (July 2012): 759–81. 134.

2.   S. Makita et al., "Influence of Mild-to-Moderate Alcohol Consumption on Cardiovascular Diseases in Men from the General Population," *Atherosclerosis* 24, no. 1 (September 2012): 222–27.

3. M. Jimenez et al., "Alcohol Consumption and Risk of Stroke in Women," *Stroke* 43, no. 4 (April 2012): 939–45.

4. Steven Reinberg, "Even in Middle Age, Starting Drink May Lower Heart Risks," accessed April 7, 2008, www.businessweek.com/print/lifestyle/content/healthday/613342.html.

5. Salynn Boyles, "Wine, Fat Intake Linked to Breast Cancer," accessed April 7, 2008, www.webmd.com/breast-cancer/news/20040317/wine-fat-intake-breast-cancer.

6. American College of Gastroenterology, "Moderate Alcohol Consumption Is Associated with Small Intestinal Bacterial Overgrowth, Study Finds" (November 28, 2011), *ScienceDaily*, retrieved November 13, 2012, http://www.sciencedaily.com /releases/2011/10/111031114949.htm.

7. Alzheimer's Association. http://www.alz.org/aaic/releases/wed_1030 amct_overview.asp, retrieved November 2012.

8. Michael T. Murray, Joseph Pizzorno, and Lara Pizzorno, "The Condensed Encyclopedia of Healing Foods" (New York: Pocket Books Publishing 2006).

9. Russell L. Blaylock, "Health and Nutrition Secrets That Can Save Your Life" (Albuquerque: Health Press 2006), 17.

10. K. Magyar et al. "Cardioprotection by Resveratrol: A Human Clinical Trial in Patients with Stable Coronary Artery Disease," *Clinical Hemorheology Microcirculation* 50, no. 3 (2012):179–87.

11. L. M. Chu et al., "Resveratrol in the Prevention and Treatment of Coronary Artery Disease," *Current Atherosclerosis Reports* 13, no. 6 (December 2011): 439–46.

12. I. Voloshyna et al., "Resveratrol Mediates Anti-Atherogenic Effects on Cholesterol Flux in Human Macrophages and Endothelium via PPARγ and Adenosine," European Journal of Pharmacology (October 2012), pii: S0014-2999(12)00736-4.

13. American Heart Association, "Alcohol Wine and Cardiovascular Disease," accessed April 7, 2008, www.americanheartassociation.org.

14. Joseph Smith, as quoted by Joel H. Johnson, *A Voice from the Mountains* (Salt Lake City: Juvenile Instructor Office, 1881), 12.

15. Brigham Young, *Discourses of Brigham Young* selected and arranged by John A. Widstoe (Salt Lake City: The Church of Jesus Christ of Latter-day Saints), 182.

16. Victor L. Ludlow, *Principles and Practices of the Restored Gospel* (Salt Lake City: Deseret Book, 1992), 434.

17. H. Burke Peterson, ed. "Q&A: Questions and Answers" *New Era* (October 1975), 36–37.

18. Page, Linda, and Sarah Abernathy, *Healthy Healing* (Healthy Healing Inc. 2006), 123.

19. Elson M. Haas and Buck Levin, "Staying Healthy with Nutrition," *The Complete Guide to Diet and Nutritional Medicine* (Berkeley, CA: Celestial Arts Publishing, 2006).

20. Johnson S. "How Diet and Regular Soda Spoil Your Health." http://voices.yahoo.com/how-diet-regular-soda-spoils-health-10589449.html?cat=5

21. Clifford J. Stratton, "Questions and Answers," *Tambuli* (August 1980), 8.

22. A. M. Rossignol and H. Bonnlander, "Prevalence and Severity of the Premenstrual Syndrome. Effects of Foods and Beverages That Are Sweet or High in Sugar Content," *Journal of Reproductive Medicine* 36 (February 1991): 131–36.

23. S. M. Creighton and S. L. Stanton, "Caffeine: Does it Affect Your Bladder?" *British Journal of Urology* 66, no. 6 (December 1990): 613–14.

24. Scorecard: The Pollution Information Site. "Health Effects: Endocrine Toxins," accessed April 15, 2008, www.scorecard.org/chemical-profiles/summary.tcl?edf_substance_id=83-067-0#hazards.

25. M. R. Olthof et al., "Consumption of High Doses of Chlorogenic Acid Present in Coffee, or of Black Tea, Increases Plasma Total Homocysteine Concentrations in Humans," *American Journal of Clinical Nutrition* 73, no. 3 (March 2001), 532–8.

26. Environmental Protection Agency, "Ground Water and Drinking Water," accessed April 15, 2008, www.epa.gov/ogwdw/hfacts.html.

27. Abernathy, *Healthy Healing*, 592.

28. Nutrition Health Review, "Some Tea and Wine May Cause Cancer—Tannin Found in Tea and Red Wine, Linked to Esophageal Cancer, accessed April 16, 2008, www.findarticles.com/p/articles/mi_m0876/is_n56/ai_9164614.

29. Jeremy E. Kaslow, "Health Issues Associated with Coffee and Caffeine," accessed April 16, 2008, http://www.drkaslow.com/html/coffee caffeine.html.

30. Elsom M. Haas and Buck Levin, "Staying Healthy with Nutrition."

CHAPTER 3

1. California Air Resources Board, "Chemical and Physical Properties of ETS," accessed November 7, 2012, www.arb.ca.gov/toxics/ets/final report/chap7b.pdf.

2. C. J. Smith et al. "IARC Carcinogens Reported in Cigarette Mainstream Smoke and Their Calculated Log P Values," *Food and Chemical Toxicology*, 41, no. 6 (June 2003, 607–17).

3. American Cancer Society, "Cigarette Smoking," accessed April 17, 2008, http://www.cancer.org/docroot/PED/content/PED_10_2X_Cigarette_Smoking.asp?sitearea=PED.

4. U.S. Department of Health and Human Services, "Reducing the Health Consequences of Smoking: 25 Years of Progress. A Report of the Surgeon General. 1989," http://profiles.nlm.nih.gov/ps/retrieve/ResourceMetadata/NNBBXS.

5. K. Pirie et al., "The 21st Century Hazards of Smoking and Benefits of Stopping: A Prospective Study of One Million Women in the UK," *Lancet* (October 26, 2012), pii: S0140-6736(12)61720-6.

6. Authors not listed. "Still Smoking? Study Finds Quitting Has Benefits at Any Age," *Harvard Women's Health Watch* 20, no. 1 (September 2012): 8.

7. R. Doll et al., "Mortality in Relation to Smoking: 50 Years' Observations on Male British Doctors," *British Medical Journal* 328, no. 7455 (2004): 1519–27.

8. American Cancer Society, "Cigarette Smoking," accessed April 17, 2008, www.cancer.org/docroot/PED/content/PED_10_2X_Cigarette_Smoking.asp?sitearea=PED

9. Government of Saskatchewan, "What Are the Health Risks Faced by Tobacco Users?" accessed April 17, 2008, from www.health.gov.sk.ca/health-effects-tobacco.

10. G. Howe et al., "Effects of Age, Cigarette Smoking, and Other Factors on Fertility: Findings in a Large Prospective Study," *British Medical Journal (Clinical Research Edition)* 290, no. 6483 (June 8, 1985): 1697–1700.

11. D. D. Baird and A. J. Wilcox, "Cigarette Smoking Associated With Delayed Conception, *JAMA* 253, no. 20 (1985): 2979–83.

12. K. T. Shiverick and C. Salafia, "Cigarette Smoking and Pregnancy I: Ovarian, Uterine and Placental Effects," *Placenta* 20, no. 4 (May 1999): 265–72.

13. S. Cnattingius, "The Epidemiology of Smoking During Pregnancy: Smoking Prevalence, Maternal Characteristics, and Pregnancy Outcomes," *Nicotine & Tobacco Research* 6, supp. 2 (April 2004): S125–40.

14. M. J. Metzger et al., "Association of Maternal Smoking during Pregnancy with Infant Hospitalization and Mortality Due to Infectious Diseases," *Pediatric Infectious Disease Journal* (August 27, 2012). [Epub ahead of print]

15. T. Conway and T. Cronan, "Smoking, Exercise, and Physical Fitness," Preventive Medicine 21, no. 6 (November 1992): 723–34.

16. C. A. Macera et al., "Cigarette Smoking, Body Mass Index, and Physical Fitness Changes among Male Navy Personnel," *Nicotine & Tobacco Research 13*, no. 10 (October 2011): 965–71.

17. American Cancer Society, "Cigarette Smoking."

18. K. Kochanek et al., "Deaths: Final Data for 2009," *National Vital Statistics Reports* 60, no. 4 (January 2012).

19. National Center for Biotechnology Information. "Nicotine Addiction: Past and Present," accessed November 2012, http://www.ncbi.nlm.nih.gov/books/NBK53018.

20. "Smoking Cessation," http://www.smoking-cessation.org/smoking_
cessation_nicotine_addiction.asp. Retrieved November 2012.

21. University of Minnesota. "Nicotine Addiction," accessed November
2012 http://www1.umn.edu/perio/tobacco/nicaddct.html.

22. Environmental Protection Agency, "Benzo(a)pyrene," accessed April
18, 2008, www.epa.gov/pbt/pubs.htm.

23. Occupational Safety Hazard Association, "Cadmium," retrieved
October 28, 2008 www.osha.gov/SLTC/cadmium/index.html.

24. About.com, "Chemicals Found in Cigarette Smoke," accessed
April 18, 2008, quitsmoking.about.com/od/chemicalinsmoke/Chemicals_
Found_in_Cigarette_Smoke.htm.

25. American Cancer Society, "Cigarette Smoking."

26. Gregory N. Connolly et al., "Trends in Smoke Nicotine Yield and
Relationship to Design Characteristics among Popular Cigarette Brands,
Tobacco Control (2007), e5.

27. Environmental Protection Agency, "An Introduction to Indoor Air
Quality: Carbon Monoxide," accessed April 18, 2008, www.epa.gov/iaq/
co.html#sources%20of%20Carbon%20Monoxide.

28. Ibid.

29. United States Department of Labor, Occupational Safety and Health
Administration, "Ammonia," accessed April 18, 2008, www.osha.gov/dts/
chemicalsampling/data/CH_218300.html.

30. Environmental Protection Agency, "Arsenic Compounds," accessed
April 18, 2008, www.epa.gov/ttn/atw/hlthef/arsenic.html.

31. Ibid.

32. Environmental Protection Agency, "Waste Minimization," accessed
April 18, 2008, www.epa.gov/minimize/factshts/cadmium.pdf.

33. Ibid.

34. U.S. Environmental Protection Agency, "The Accelerated Phaseout of
Class I Ozone-Depleting Substances," accessed November 2012, http://www.
epa.gov/ozone/title6/phaseout/accfact.html.

35. Environmental Protection Agency, "Chloroform," accessed April 18, 2008www.epa.gov/ttn/atw/hlthef/chlorofo.html.

36. Environmental Protection Agency, "Formaldehyde," accessed April 18, 2008, from www.epa.gov/iris/subst/0419.htm.

37. Ibid.

38. T. I. Lidsky and J. S. Schneider, "Lead Neurotoxicity in Children: Basic Mechanisms and Clinical Correlates," *Brain* 126, pt. 1 (January 2003): 5–19.

39. Environmental Protection Agency, "Lead in Paint, Dust, and Soil: Basic Information," accessed April 22, 2008, www.epa.gov/lead/pubs/leadinfo.htm.

40. Environmental Protection Agency, "Vinyl Chloride," accessed April 18, 2008, www.epa.gov/ttn/atw/hlthef/vinylchl.html.

41. American Cancer Society, "Secondhand Smoke," accessed April 22, 2008, http://www.cancer.org/docroot/PED/content/PED_10_2X_Secondhand_Smoke-Clean_Indoor_Air.asp.

42. California Environmental Protection Agency, "Identification of Environmental Tobacco Smoke as a Toxic Air Contaminant," Executive Summary, June 2005.

43. Ibid.

44. Ibid.

45. M. A. Schuster, T. Franke, and C. B. Pham, "Smoking Patterns of Household Members and Visitors in Homes with Children in the United States," *Archives of Pediatric Adolescent Medicine* 156, (November 2002): 1094–1100.

46. Surgeon General, U.S. Department of Health and Human Services, "The Health Consequences of Involuntary Exposure to Tobacco Smoke: A Report of the Surgeon General, 6 major conclusions of the surgeon general report," accessed April 22, 2008, from http://www.surgeongeneral.gov/library/secondhandsmoke/factsheets/factsheet6.html.

47. Campaign for Tobacco-Free Kids, "Toll of Tobacco in the United States," accessed November 2012, https://www.tobaccofreekids.org/facts_issues/toll_us.

48. American Cancer Society, "Smokeless Tobacco and How to Quit," accessed April 17, 2008, from http://www.cancer.org/docroot/PED_10_13X_ Quitting_Smokeless_Tobacco.asp?sitearea=PED.

49. National Cancer Institute, "Smokeless Tobacco and Cancer: Questions and Answers," accessed April 17, 2008, www.cancer.gov/ cancertopics/factsheet/tobacco/smokeless.

50. American Cancer Society, "Smokeless Tobacco and How to Quit," accessed April 17, 2008, http://www.cancer.org/docroot/PED_10_13X_ Quitting_Smokeless_Tobacco.asp?sitearea=PED.

51. Science Watch, "No Help for the Hungry" (April 28, 1981), accessed April 22, 2008, http://query.nytimes.com/gst/fullpage.html?sec=technology&res=9B07E3DA1638F93BA15757C0A967948260.

52. George Albert Smith, Conference Report (April 1918), 40.

CHAPTER 4

1. The Free Dictionary: Medical Dictionary, "Constitution," accessed April 23, 2008, http://medical-dictionary.thefreedictionary.com/constitution. See also Merriam-Webster Dictionary, "Constitution," www.merriam-webster. com/dictionary/constitution, retrieved April 23, 2008.

2. Merriam-Webster Dictionary, "Ordain," accessed November 2012, http://www.merriam-webster.com/dictionary/ordain.

3. Avicenna Natural Products, "Hippocrates 400–377 B.C.," accessed November 2012, http://www.avicennanatural.com/history/ hippocrates-400-377-b-c/.

4. Brigham Young, "Journal History: August 19, 1846" (Salt Lake City: Church History Library).

5. Brigham Young, as reported by David W. Evans, "Discourse by President Brigham Young, August 13, 1875," *Journal of Discourses* 18:71, jod. mrm.org/18/70.

6. Spencer W. Kimball, "President Kimball Speaks Out on Administration to the Sick," *Tambuli* (August 1982), 34.

7.   J. Lazarou, B. Pomeranz, and P. N. Corey, "Incidence of Adverse Drug Reactions in Hospitalized Patients. A Meta-Analysis of Prospective Studies," *Journal of the American Medical Association* 279 (April 1998): 1200–5.

8.   Dan Hurley, "Diet Supplements and Safety: Some Disquieting Data," *New York Times*, January 16, 2007; corrected article February 6, 2007, www.nytimes.com/2007/01/16/health/16diet.html?pagewanted=all.

9.   Ibid.

10. Ibid.

11. Ibid.

12. Ellen Nolte and C. Martin McKee, "Measuring the Health of Nations: Updating an Earlier Analysis," *Health Affairs* 27, no. 1 (January/February 2008): 58–71.

13. Central Intelligence Agency, "The World Fact Book 2008: Rank Order of Life Expectancy at Birth," www. cia.gov/library/publications/the-world-fact-book/rankorder/2102rank.html.

14. K. Linde, M. M. Berner, and L. Kriston, "St. John's Wort for Major Depression," *Cochrane Database of Systematic Reviews*, 2009 (4): CD000448.

15. Mayo Clinic, "St. John's Wort," accessed November 2012, http://www.mayoclinic.com/health/st-johns-wort/NS_patient-stjohnswort/DSECTION=evidence.

16. Mayo Clinic, "St. John's Wort," accessed April 25, 2008, www.mayoclinic.com/health/st-johns-wort/NS_patient-stjohnswort.

17. Mayo Clinic, "Monoamine Oxidase Inhibitors," accessed April 25, 2008, www.mayoclinic.com/health/maois/MH00072.

18. Aaron Catlin et al., "National Health Spending in 2005: The Slowdown Continues," *Health Affairs* 26, no. 1 (2006), 142–53.

19. California Health Care Foundation, "Health care costs 101: – 2005" (March 2, 2005), accessed April 25, 2008, www.chcf.org.

20. Ibid.

21. Catlin et al., "National Health Spending in 2005: The Slowdown Continues."

CHAPTER 5

1. L. D'Elia et al., "Potassium Intake, Stroke, and Cardiovascular Disease: A Meta-Analysis of Prospective Studies," *Journal of the American College of Cardiology* 57, no. 10 (March 2011): 1210–19.

2. L. Brown et al., "Cholesterol-Lowering Effects of Dietary Fiber: A <eta-analysis. American Journal of Clinical Nutrition 69, no. 1 (January 1999): 30–42.

3. M. Higgins, "Color Me Healthy: Enjoying Fruits and Vegetables Fact Sheet," August 2004.

4. North Dakota State University, "Publications," accessed November 2012, http://www.ag.ndsu.edu/pubs/yf/foods/fn595w.htm.

5. Joy Bauer, "Health Benefits of Healthy Vegetables," accessed November 2012, http://www.joybauer.com/food-articles/starchy-vegetables. aspx.

6. F. He, C. Nowson, M. Lucas, and G. MacGregor, "Increased Consumption of Fruits and Vegetables is Related to a Reduced Risk of Coronary Heart Disease: Meta-Analysis of Cohort Studies," *Journal of Human Hypertension* 21 (September 2007): 717–28.

7. Ancel Keys, "Seven Countries: A Multivariate Analysis of Death and Coronary Heart Disease), *Annals of Internal Medicine* 93, no. 5 (November 1980): 786–87.

8. F. He et al., "Fruit and Vegetable Consumption and Stroke: Meta-Analysis of Cohort Studies," *Lancet* 367 (January 2006): 320–26.

9. U.S. Department of Agriculture, "Why Is It Important to Eat Vegetables?" accessed April 30, 2008, www.mypyramid.gov/pyramid/ vegetables_why.html.

10. G. Block, B. Patterson, and A. Subar A. "Fruit, Vegetables, and Cancer Prevention: A Review of the Epidemiological Evidence," *Nutrition and Cancer* 18, no. 1 (1992): 1–29.

11. Medline Plus, "Portion Size," accessed November 2012, http://www. nlm.nih.gov/medlineplus/ency/patientinstructions/000337.htm.

12. University of Michigan Intergrative Medicine, "Healing Foods Pyramid," accessed November 2012, http://www.med.umich.edu/umim/food-pyramid/fruits_and_vegetables.htm.

13. N. I. Krinsky, J. T. Landrum, R. A. Bone, "Biological Mechanisms of the Protective Role of Lutein and Zeaxanthin in the Eye," *Annual Review of Nutrition* 23 (February 2003), 171–201.

14. S. M. Moeller, P. F. Jacques, and J. B. Blumberg, "The Potential Role of Dietary Xanthophylls in Cataract and Age-Related Macular Degeneration. Journal of the American College of Nutrition 19, no. 5 supp. (October 2000): 522S–527S.

15. U.S. Department of Agriculture, "Why Is It Important to Eat Vegetables?"

16. Ibid.

17. C. Hernandez and M. Hernandez, "The Basic Approach to Good Health: Acid/Akaline Balance in the Body," accessed November 2012, http://www.pacificnaturopathic.com/articles/acid_alkaline_balance_in_the_body.html.

18. J. Kim, G. K. Jayaprakasha, and B. S. Patil, "Limonoids and Their Anti-Proliferative and Anti-Aromatase Properties in Human Breast Cancer Cells," *Food & Function* (November 1, 2012). [Epub ahead of print]

19. K. Park et al., "Induction of the Cell Cycle Arrest and Apoptosis by Flavonoids Isolated from Korean Citrusaurantium L. in Non-Small-Cell Lung Cancer Cells," *Food Chemistry* 135, no. 4 (December 2012): 2728–35.

20. T. Hirano et al., "Citrus Flavone Tangeretin Inhibits Leukaemic HL-60 Cell Growth Partially through Induction of Apoptosis with Less Cytotoxicity on Normal Lymphocytes," British Journal of Cancer 72, no. 6 (December 1995): 1380–88.

21. P. Qiu et al., "The Inhibitory Effects of 5-hydroxy-3,6,7,8,3',4'-hexamethoxyflavone on Human Colon Cancer Cells," *Molecular Nutrition & Food Research* 55, no. 10 (October 2011): 1523-32.

22. Elson M. Haas and Buck Levin, "Staying Healthy with Nutrition," *The Complete Guide to Diet and Nutrition* (Berkeley, CA: Celestial Arts Publishing, 2006).

CHAPTER 6

1.   Mark Bittman, "Rethinking the Meat-Guzzler," *New York Times*, January 27, 2008.

2.   Ibid.

3.   Ibid.

4.   J. M. Genkinger and A. Koushik, "Meat Consumption and Cancer Risk," *PLoS Medicine* 4, no. 12 (December 2007): e345, www.plosmedicine.org/article/info%3Adoi%2F10.1371%2Fjournal.pmed.0040345.

5.   Ibid.

6.   L. Aston, J. Smith, and J. Powles, "Impact of a Reduced Red and Processed Meat Dietary Pattern on Disease Risks and Greenhouse Gas Emissions in the UK: A Modelling Study, *BMJ Open* 2 (2012): e001072

7.   Micha R et al., "Red and Processed Meat Consumption and Risk of Incident Coronary Heart Disease, Stroke, and Diabetes Mellitus," *Circulation* 121 (2010): 2271–83.

8.   A. A. Nanji and S. W. French, "Relationship between Pork Consumption and Cirrhosis," *Lancet* 1, no. 8430 (March 1985): 681–83.

9.   W. Connor, "Importance of N–3 Fatty Acids in Health and Disease," *American Journal of Clinical Nutrition* 71, no. 1 (January 2000): 171S-175S.

10.   B. M. Yashodhara, "Omega-3 Fatty Acids: A Comprehensive Review of Their Role in Health and Disease," Postgraduate Medical Journal 85, no. 1000 (February 2009): 84–90.

11.   McDonald's Corporation, "Nutrition," accessed October 16, 2008, www.nutrition.mcdonalds.com/bagamcmeal/nutrition_facts.html, retrieved October 16, 2008.

12.   Burger King Corporation, "Menu Nutrition," accessed October 16, 2008, www.bk.com/en/us/menu-nutrition/index.html.

13.   Livestrong, "The Daily Plate," accessed October 16, 2008, www.thedailyplate.com.

14.   T. C. Campbell, T. M. Campbell, *The China Study*, (Dallas: Benbella Books, 2004).

15. R. Cohen, *Milk, the Deadly Poison*, 1st ed. (Los Angeles: Argus Publishing, 1997).

16. K. Sonneville et al., "Vitamin D, Calcium, and Dairy Intakes and Stress Fractures Among Female Adolescents," *Archives of Pediatric & Adolescent Medicine* 166, no. 7 (July 2012): 595–600.

17. June M. Chan and Edward L. Giocannucci, "Dairy Products, Calcium, and Vitamin D and the Risk of Prostate Cancer," *Epidemiology Reviews* 23 (2001): 87–92.

18. Y. T. Tsai, P. C. Cheng, and T. M. Pan, "The Immunomodulatory Effects of Lactic Acid Bacteria for Improving Immune Functions and Benefits," *Applied Microbiology and Biotechnology* 96, no. 4 (November 2012): 853–62.

19. A. Hakansson A and G. Molin, "Gut Microbiota and Inflammation," *Nutrients* 3, no. 6 (June 2011): 637–82.

20. Ezra Taft Benson E, "In His Steps," *Ensign*, September 1988, 2.

21. World Health Organization, "International Day for the Eradication of Poverty," http://www.un.org/esa/socdev/poverty/images/IDEP_flyer.pdf , Accessed November 2012.

22. FAO Newsroom, "Livestock's Long Shadow—Environmental Issues and Options," accessed October 15, 2008, www.fao.org/newsroom/en/news/2006/1000448/index.html.

23. Ibid.

24. Ibid.

CHAPTER 7

1. Ezra Taft Benson, "Do Not Despair," *Tambuli*, March 1987, 2.

2. Penn State, "Whole Grain Diets Lower Risk of Chronic Disease, Study Shows," *ScienceDaily* (February 11, 2008), accessed November 14, 2012, from http://www.sciencedaily.com /releases/2008/02/080205161231.htm.

3. J. P. Karl and E. Saltzman E., "The Role of Whole Grains in Body Weight Regulation," *Advanced Nutrition* 3, no. 5 (September 2012): 697–707.

4.   The World's Healthiest Foods, "Fiber from Whole Grains and Fruit Protective against Breast Cancer," accessed October 22, 2008, www.whfoods.com.

5.   Ibid.

6.   M. J. McCann et al., "Enterolactone Restricts the Proliferation of the LNCaP Human Prostate Cancer Cell Line In Vitro," *Molecular Nutrition and Research* 52 (April 2008): 567–80.

7.   J. Peterson et al., "Dietary Lignans: Physiology and Potential for Cardiovascular Disease Risk Reduction," Nutrition Reviews 68, no. 10 (October 2010): 571–603.

8.   K. Buck et al., "Meta-Analyses of Lignans and Enterolignans in Relation to Breast Cancer Risk," American Journal of Clinical Nutrition 92, no. 1 (July 2010): 141–53.

9.   P. L. Horn-Ross et al., "Phytoestrogen Intake and Endometrial Cancer Risk," *Journal of the National Cancer Institute* 95, no. 15. (August 2003): 1158–64.

10.   S. J. Bhathena and M. T. Velasquez, "Beneficial Role of Dietary Phytoestrogens in Obesity and Diabetes," American Journal of Clinical Nutrition 76, no. 6 (December 2002): 1191–201.

11.   N. McKeown et al., "Whole-Grain Intake is Favorably Associated with Metabolic Risk Factors for Type 2 Diabetes and Cardiovascular Disease in the Framingham Offspring Study," American Journal of Clinical Nutrition 76, no. 2 (August 2002): 390–98.

12.   J. E. Gerich, "Clinical Significance, Pathogenesis, and Management of Postprandial Hyperglycemia," *Archives of Internal Medicine* 163, no. 11 (June 2003): 1306–16.

13.   A. Ceriello et al., "Evidence for an Independent and Cumulative Effect of Postprandial Hypertriglyceridemia and Hyperglycemia on Endothelial Dysfunction and Oxidative Stress Generation," *Circulation* 106, no. 10 (September 2002):1211-8.

14.   J. H. O'Keefe and D. S. Bell, "Postprandial Hyperglycemia/ Hyperlipidemia (Postprandial Dysmetabolism) is a Cardiovascular Risk Factor," American Journal of Cardiology 100, no. 5 (September 2007): 899–904.

15. Food and Agriculture Organization, "Wheat in the World," http://www.fao.org/docrep/006/y4011e/y4011e04.htm, accessed November 2012.

16. Ezra Taft Benson, "In His Steps," *Ensign*, September 1988, 2.

17. The World's Healthiest Foods, "Fiber from Whole Grains and Fruit Protective against Breast Cancer."

18. K. J. Carpenter, "The Relationship of Pellagra to Corn and the Low Availability of Niacin in Cereals," *Experientia Supplement* 44 (1983): 197–222.

19. Kafui Adom and Rui Hai Liu, "Antioxidant Activity of Grains," Journal of Agriculture and Food Chemistry 50 (2002)6182–87.

20. J. D. Ribaya-Mercado and J. B. Blumberg, "Lutein and Zeaxanthin and Their Potential Roles in Disease Prevention," *Journal of the American College of Nutrition* 23 (6 supp.): 567S–587S.

21. R. A. Othman, M. H. Moghadasian, and P. J. Jones, "Cholesterol-Lowering Effects of Oat β-glucan," *Nutrition Review* 69, no. 6 (June 2011): 299–309.

22. K. A. Harris and P. M. Kris-Etherton, "Effects of Whole Grains on Coronary Heart Disease Risk," *Current Atherosclerosis Reports* 12, no. 6 (November 2010): 368–76.

23. M. Meydani, "Potential Health Benefits of Avenanthramides of Oats," Nutrition Reviews 67, no. 12 (December 2009): 731–35.

24. H. Bays et al., "Reduced Viscosity Barley β-Glucan versus Placebo: A Randomized Controlled Trial of the Effects on Insulin Sensitivity for Individuals at Risk for Diabetes Mellitus," *Nutrition & Metabolism* (Lond.) 8 August 2011): 58.

25. P. Kallio et al., "Dietary Carbohydrate Modification Induces Alterations in Gene Expression in Abdominal Subcutaneous Adipose Tissue in Persons with the Metabolic Syndrome: The FUNGENUT Study," *American Journal of Clinical Nutrition* 85, no. 5 (May 2007): 1417–27.

CHAPTER 8

1. Gordon B. Hinckley, "Come and Partake," *Ensign*, May 1986, 49.

2.   Joseph Fielding Smith, *Church History and Modern Revelation*, 1 (Salt Lake City: The Church of Jesus Christ of Latter-day Saints), 383.

3.   Joseph Fielding Smith, *Improvement Era*, February 1956, 78–79.

4.   Ray M. Merrill, "Life Expectancy among LDS and Non-LDS in Utah, 2004," accessed November 11, 2008, www.demographic-research.org/volumes/vol10/3/.

5.   J. L. Lyon, K. Gardner, and R. E. Gress, "Cancer Incidence among Mormons and Non-Mormons in Utah, 1971–85," *Cancer Causes Control* 5 (March 1994): 149–56, accessed November 4, 2008, www.ncbi.nlm.nih.gov/pubmed/8167262.

APPENDIX B

1.   Michael T. Murray, Joseph Pizzorno, and Lara Pizzorno, *The Condensed Encyclopedia of Healing Foods*, (New York: Pocket Books Publishing, 2006).

2.   Elson M. Haas and Buck Levin, *Staying Healthy with Nutrition: The Complete Guide to Diet and Nutritional Medicine* (Berkeley, CA: Celestial Arts Publishing), 2006.

3.   Ibid.

4.   Laurie Deutsch Mozian, *Foods That Fight Disease: A Simple Guide to Using and Understanding Phytonutrients to Protect and Enhance Your Health* (New York: Avery Publishing), 2000.

5.   F. Shahidi, "Antinutrients and Phytochemicals in Food," American Chemical Society, 1997.

Index

S

T

V

W

Y

About *the* Author

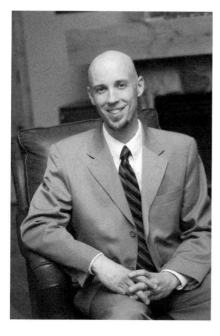

Scott Johnson spent most of his childhood in Orem, Utah, where he gained a love for writing. Recognizing his potential at a young age, his teachers and family encouraged him to explore his developing writing talents.

A health challenge propelled him to study natural health and the Word of Wisdom intensely. He graduated from college with a doctorate in naturopathy. Today, he shares his knowledge of health through more than 200 published health and fitness articles. He lives a healthy lifestyle and encourages others to do so by example.

Scott, his wife, and four children reside in Utah County where they enjoy the mountains and outdoors. Scott is regularly asked for health guidance by neighbors, friends, family, and acquaintances and enjoys teaching others how to support the body's innate ability to heal through natural methods.